Jerome Sachs
Fred Newdom

Clinical W
and Social Action
An Integrative Approach

Pre-publication
REVIEWS, .
COMMENTARIES,
EVALUATIONS . . .

"*Clinical Work and Social Action* is an important new tool for helping social welfare practitioners better understand the meaning of their work. By presenting political and educational theorists in an accessible way, Sachs and Newdom give frontline clinicians a chance to understand the potential of their work both for help and for harm. They don't give up on the possibility for social workers to make a positive difference, but they carefully demonstrate how 'contradictory' the effort is, and how important it is that direct service workers at all levels adopt a critical, nonhierarchical stance toward all aspects of their practice.

Sachs and Newdom make an especially important contribution to social work education by giving extensive and concrete examples of how teachers can help students face the contradictions in their work and collectively devise strategies for working effectively with people as allies, not as elite professionals. Since Bertha Capen Reynolds wrote about social work teaching more than fifty years ago, no other writers have done this better."

Ann Withorn, PhD
Professor of Social Policy,
College of Public
and Community Service,
University of Massachusetts, Boston

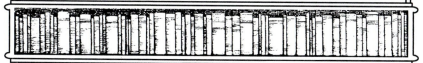

"**T**his book was developed from a course that the authors have taught for several years at the Smith College School for Social Work. As a result, it is full of practical suggestions and guidelines for social work educators who want to integrate clinical work with the possibility of social action and change. The volume is an excellent text for undergraduate and graduate social work practice courses. It offers a unique blend of theoretical frameworks, including phenomenology, Freudian thought, symbolic interaction, and critical theory, that can help students to understand the psychosocial context of social work practice and method.

Students will find the book helpful because of the many practical applications. The authors are careful to keep their ideas grounded in the pragmatics of everyday social work clinical practice, and the book is replete with examples and applications. It also contains a chapter describing how to apply their ideas in the classroom and how to engage students in a seemingly conflictual way that encourages personal reflection and growth. They describe how the process they use has affected them personally, leading to personal growth and change. Throughout, Sachs and Newdom take great pains to point out and clarify practice principles and contradictions. At the same time, the book is engaging and personal and will benefit many students, practitioners, and educators."

Keith M. Kilty, PhD
Professor,
College of Social Work,
Ohio State University,
Columbus, Ohio

"**J**ust in time for the next millennium come Sachs and Newdom with a wholly fresh look at social work. *Clinical Work and Social Action* unites two threads, proving that their historical tension can be resolved. It illustrates a new way both to improve clients' lives and rectify social, political, and economic ills. A much-needed uniting of social work values, theories, and practice for action."

Josephine Nieves, MSW, PHD
Executive Director,
National Association of Social Workers

Clinical Work
and Social Action
An Integrative Approach

Clinical Work and Social Action
An Integrative Approach

Jerome Sachs
Fred Newdom

The Haworth Press
New York • London • Oxford

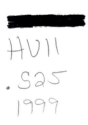

The Haworth Press, Inc., 10 Alice Street, Binghamton, NY 13904-1580

Cover design by Marylouise E. Doyle.

Material cited from Hasenfeld, Y. (1987), "Power in social work"; and Mead, G. H. (1934), *Mind, Self, and Society,* reprinted with permission from The University of Chicago Press.

Library of Congress Cataloging-in-Publication Data

Sachs, Jerome.
    Clinical work and social action : an integrative approach / Jerome Sachs, Fred Newdom.
       p.   cm.
    Includes bibliographical references and index.
    ISBN 0-7890-0278-7 (alk. paper) — ISBN 0-7890-0279-5 (soft cover)
    1. Social work education. 2. Social action—Study and teaching. I. Newdom, Fred. II. Title.

HV11.S25 1999
361.3'2—dc21
                                                          99-016076
                                                              CIP

To our wives, Nancy and Susan,
and children, Katie and Eric

ABOUT THE AUTHORS

Jerome Sachs, DSW, is Associate Professor at Smith College School for Social Work, where he teaches in the practice and human behavior and the social environment sequences. Dr. Sachs has written articles and presented at conferences on topics that include play and psychoanalysis, work with a group of homeless people, the phenomenology of social work practice, and clinical work and social action. In 1992 he produced two hour-long videos on the lives of a homeless man and a homeless woman. Before going to Smith College in 1987, Dr. Sachs worked with street gangs, was a group worker and community organizer in settlement houses, and practiced and supervised psychoanalysis. He also taught social work, sociology, and psychoanalysis in New York City. For the last twelve years, he has been involved with issues of rural homelessness and welfare rights. In addition, Dr. Sachs is a member of the steering committee of the Bertha Capen Reynolds Society.

Fred Newdom, ACSW, is Professor of ProAct, an Albany, New York, consulting firm specializing in advocacy and organizational development services. He also teaches courses in social policy at the Smith College School for Social Work in Massachusetts and other schools. Mr. Newdom also has served as chair of the Board of New York State NARAL (National Abortion and Reproductive Rights Action League) and is currently chair of the Bertha Capen Reynolds Society, a national organization of progressive workers in the human services. His advocacy work has included work with AIDS organizations, legislative and organizing projects related to tax policy, lobbying for the WIC program, and working for decent welfare reform. He was Executive Director of the New York State chapter of the National Association of Social Workers (NASW) and chaired NASW's Committee on Peace and Social Justice.

Dr. Sachs and Mr. Newdom collectively bring over seventy years of casework, group work, and social justice to the writing of this book.

CONTENTS

Acknowledgments

We owe debts to the many people who have helped us give birth to this book. First and foremost, we thank the students who asked us to develop and teach the course on which the book is based. We are indebted to all students who took this course, for their courage and generosity as they shared their ideas, feelings, and practice. They challenged us with questions and comments that forced us out of the boxes we inhabit. The book would not be as it is but for the permission they granted us to use the work they shared with each other and with us.

Many colleagues reviewed various parts of the manuscript. We especially want to thank Joel Blau, who thankfully, could not resist going through the entire manuscript even as he was working on his own book. His ideas and comments and our answers to his questions are everywhere. We are also indebted to Ira Shor, who met with us at an early stage, made helpful comments, and assuaged our insecurity by telling us that he thought we had a contribution to make.

We also want to thank those who helped us and/or encouraged us along the way: Mimi Abramovitz, Ann Withorn, Katherine Keating, Lucy Fox, Jonathan Levy, Fred Swan, and Muriel Poulin. We apologize to anyone we may inadvertently have left out. You know who you are and we ask for your forgiveness in advance. It needs to be said that the final responsibility for the book rests with us.

We should like to thank our publisher, The Haworth Press, and particularly, Carlton Munson, the series editor. Acknowledgment also needs to go to the editorial staff at The Haworth Press who helped us through various stages of the publishing process.

Jerry Sachs would like to thank Smith College School for Social Work for the sabbatical time he received during the 1997-1998 school year and the Brown Foundation for the grant he received from the Clinical Research Institute of Smith College School for

Social Work. This book would have taken more time and a greater personal toll if not for this support.

To my family I give my love for their tolerance, gentle pushing, and good humor. My daughter Katie's passion for social justice and her willingness to act on her own values reinforces and gives meaning to the work I do. My wife, Nancy Kirschner Sachs, who has found her own passion in creating sculptural pottery even as she continues to advocate for clients in her clinical work, receives singular blessings for her encouragement, support of my political activities, and helpful editing of several chapters. (JS)

I want to offer my heartfelt thanks to my family for seeing through the process of writing this book. My son Eric's love for and faith in me has provided precious support for pursuing my own dreams, as he pursues his. Most of all, I want to thank my wife, Susan Faulkner, for her love, comradeship, encouragement, and the inspiration that her example provided me. Susan's completion of her dissertation made it possible for me to have hope that this book, too, could be finished. She has been my muse and guiding spirit throughout this effort. (FN)

Chapter 1

Introduction

This book grew out of discussions with students training to be clinicians at Smith College School for Social Work. They valued their psychodynamic clinical training but recognized that it omitted the element of social action that had attracted many of them to the profession. They were disturbed that advocacy and social action, asserted in the profession's values and ethics, were generally absent and sometimes discouraged in the training they received, and that their training was dichotomized. This historical dichotomy between clinical work and social action, between the approaches of Mary Richmond and Jane Addams, continues today in social work schools and social agencies, despite lip service to the contrary.

Our students identified the contradiction (a central concept for us) between their own and the profession's values, theories, and practice. We shared and were encouraged by their concerns. At their urging, we designed an advanced elective course, given for the first time in 1992, that attempted to resolve the contradictions we were all experiencing. This book, including its title, grows out of that course.

A social work student placed at a family service agency in a major city records a typical clinical encounter (see Appendix A for a full transcript of the process recording):

Mary, the client: Let's see. Where to begin? I'm really concerned about my boyfriend [Larry]. I don't know where to start. I guess I'm mostly concerned about the fact that he's gotten a hold of a handgun and, well, he's been acting pretty strange lately.

1

Worker*: So, you're concerned about what he might want to do with a handgun?

Mary: Yeah. It was weird. Things have not been going well for him.

(Client proceeds to tell that her boyfriend has lost his job, and as a result will have to quit school because work was subsidizing his coursework. Although the client has been distancing from this boyfriend for the past two months, and they have had fights, she felt sorry for him and went to his apartment to console him on Saturday.)

Most reasonably, the worker's first response was a question related to the client's personal safety. This intervention was supported both by the supervisor in her marginal notes and, subsequently, our class's beginning discussion about the case. All reasonable clinicians would want to engage the real potential for danger to the client. All good clinicians, we would expect, would see this as necessary and many, if not most, would see this as sufficient. The client's safety needs to be assured.

This approach, however, omits a major concern expressed by the client in her first statement. Specifically, she was "really concerned about my boyfriend." The concern she expressed was both about his possession of a handgun and about his well-being. He lost his job and had to leave school. To respond to the full range of client concerns would require being open to larger social and economic issues such as layoffs, domestic violence, social class, unequal access to education, and availability of handguns, among others. The worker would have to engage the client in discussion of both the social and individual issues the client raised. These discussions would move us to work on individual and social action levels simultaneously: to bridge the false dichotomy between clinical work and social action.

Our objective is to develop a model of practice that integrates clinical work and social action for human service workers. Practice

---

* Most of our students come into the class labeling themselves as therapists. We make a point about this and emphasize the use of "worker" as our preferred label. This is done to stress identification with the role of *social worker* and the political meanings of these two words.

takes place where intrapersonal, interpersonal, and institutional forces come together. The interaction between and among these forces precipitates effects within workers, clients, agencies, and other institutions and organizations that are connected to the process of work. A worker's awareness of the personal and institutional forces will direct him or her to the structures that need to be changed to accommodate the needs of particular clients. For example, an agency's intake structure may encourage or discourage a person's willingness to become a client. This would depend on the "goodness of fit" (Germain and Gitterman, 1980) between a client's needs and personality and the agency's structures and procedures.

Though we would reverse the order, we agree with those scholars who have emphasized that a practice model seeking to affect the psychosocial interface ought to be "under the conscious guidance of knowledge and values" (Gordon, 1962, p. 5).

No practice is value free. In all clinical encounters, there are a multitude of possible interventions. The choice of intervention a given worker makes reflects many complex forces. These include the worker's values, theories, experiences, training, feelings, and ideas as well as an agency's goals, structures, and policies. In addition, the needs and interests of funding sources, including third party payers, licensing bodies, and policymakers have an impact. Finally, other social forces including racism, classism, heterosexism and sexism are in the mix that influences a worker's interventions.

Similarly, no theory is value free. Theoretical ideas reflect prevailing social, economic, and political interests. The current dichotomy between clinical work and social action serves particular institutional interests. Individualizing problems and solutions deflects attention from wider social forces as a cause of personal and social problems (Mills, 1961). For example, homelessness is blamed on mental illness, substance abuse, or personal failure rather than declining funding for affordable housing and lack of employment (Blau, 1992).

Maintaining the dichotomy between clinical work and social action is a practice that maintains the politics of the status quo. It focuses the worker's and client's attention on a client's private troubles (Mills, 1961). Bridging the dichotomy develops a practice that includes the possibility of social change. It focuses a worker's and a client's attention simultaneously on the client's (and worker's) inner world as well as how the inner world reflects social institutions (Fanon, 1967). This connection points to possibilities for linking social action and clinical work. It also opens the door to changing the social institutions and structure of a society. For example, in the model that we propose, an unemployed highly skilled client who could not pay an agency's fee would not immediately be seen as "resistant." He or she more properly would first be seen as just not having money. The worker would need to consider problems in the political economy that foster internalized oppression, diminishing the client's self-esteem, and arousing anger against an agency that defines the effects of social issues as a personal weakness or deficit.

Rarely has the psychosocial interface actually been the central focus of values, theory, and practice. Rein and White (1981) noted that knowledge, and we add values, rather than informing practice, is used primarily as a justification for practice. "[Values], knowledge, and practice are split." For example, "burnout" and "hard-to-reach client" are concepts that deflect attention away from racist and classist values as well as social issues that cry out for deep reflection and action. In a model that truly takes account of these issues, this reflection would call forth strategies of social action as part of clinical work.

We need both a clearly defined value base that will inform the vision, mission, goals, and direction of practice and a theory or integrated set of theories that will provide the knowledge a practitioner needs to do good work—clinically and politically. A practice model and/or the practice of any practitioner can then be observed to conform to or conflict with these values and theories. Finally, a method to observe and address contradictions must be an integral part of this model.

It is our conviction that the theories we choose to inform our practice must be those which are consistent with our values and that our practice must be consistent with both our values and our theory. We underscore this point because, to the best of our knowledge, current practice theories express a commitment to this formulation but have not carried it out.

What follows is a summary of the values and knowledge that are central to informing our practice model. We offer several key ideas and concepts, many of which highlight contradictions in work with clients and classroom teaching. This will provide the context for the in-depth discussions and analyses of theoretical issues and case material that will be presented in this book.

VALUES

The central values we propose to direct and guide practice are as follows:

- *Self-determination* of communities, groups, families, and individuals. This implies both knowledge of one's world and the means to act on it (Freire, 1989a). The clinical encounter is a setting in which this ought to be realized.
- *Economic and political justice.* It is our contention that social justice, a term used with great regularity, if not clarity, in the human services, is meaningless without political and economic justice. Our model for economic and political justice draws heavily on politically progressive formulations.
- A belief and commitment to *dialogical praxis* (Freire, 1989a). This is a process of action and reflection between two Subjects (people who accord each other equal worth) who meet to examine and transform their world.

These values reflect a commitment to work where psychological and social forces interact. They are rooted in ideas that value raising people's consciousness about themselves and the social institutions that affect their lives. They demand the exploration of unconscious processes at the intrapsychic level (Freud, 1915/1963c) as well as the processes that produce false consciousness about race, class, gender, sexual orientation, and ethnic issues at the social-institutional level.

Obviously, there are other important values, which have a place in practice. These generally can be subsumed under one or another of the values noted above. For example, we see confidentiality as part of self-determination, and nondiscrimination included under economic and political justice as well as self-determination.

THEORETICAL KNOWLEDGE

Our model integrates phenomenological (Husserl, 1967; Schutz, 1967; Luckman, 1978), psychoanalytic (Freud, 1900; Langs, 1981;

Fanon, 1967), symbolic interaction (Mead, 1934), critical theory (Horkheimer, 1937; Wiggershaus; 1994; Roderick, 1986; Marcuse, 1966, 1969), and their modern derivatives. These are the primary theoretical lenses we have chosen to use for analyzing the structures and dynamic processes that interact in practice. The selective use and integration of these theories will guarantee a close reflective inspection of practice in a way that is compatible with our values:

- *Phenomenology* forces the observer's attention to the structures and processes, both psychological and sociological, that interact constantly among individuals, families, groups, communities, and the institutional context that surrounds them.
- *Psychoanalytic* concepts and ideas provide a powerful tool to analyze unconscious structures and motivational processes of the individual.
- *Symbolic interaction theory* provides an understanding of the ways in which the contents of the social world are internalized by the individual, including the internalization of the social world into the individual's unconscious.
- *Critical theory* provides a powerful analysis of the social structure and its effects on the lives and consciousness of individuals, groups, families, and communities.

Integrating and using the seemingly disparate ideas of such a wide range of theorists and theoretical formulations need not dissuade us. It can actually facilitate a fuller understanding of the interaction between psychological and social forces. For example, Smelser (1973) noted:

some formal parallels in the thought of Karl Marx and Sigmund Freud. Both their theories concern a system that maintains an equilibrium-in-tension between conflicting forces. For Marx, the tension is expressed at bottom in contradictions between the mode of production and the social relations of production, but manifests itself in the antagonism between two classes. For Freud the tension is between instinctual impulses (the id), and various personality establishments engaged in the management and control of these impulses. . . . Both theorists stress, moreover, that the main strategy for control is a form of repression, political-economic in one case and psychological in the other. Furthermore, in each case the repressive forces are buttressed by a number of ancillary devices that lead to distortions of reality and consciousness. For Marx, one of the main functions of religion, philosophy, morality, and so on is to disguise the true interests of the workers, and to contribute to a false consciousness in them; for Freud various mechanisms of defense such as projection, isolation, rationalization, and displacement distort the true nature of the impulses and obscure them from the individual. For Marx, moreover, the structure of society results from the efforts of the dominant class to save itself from the destructive impact of societal contradictions; for Freud, the structure of the personality (character traits, symptoms, and so forth) is geared in large measure to saving the individual from the destructive impact of his [sic] inner conflicts. Finally, for both authors, freedom from repression is gained by an expansion of awareness (consciousness) of the conflicts besetting the system. (pp. xxxiii-xxxiv)

PRACTICE, PRAXIS, AND CONTRADICTIONS

In the language of grounded theory (Glaser and Strauss, 1967), the fit and workability between values, theory, and practice should constantly be examined. A practice model is needed that identifies and engages the contradictions between values and theories which direct, guide, and inform practice, and the actual practice which takes place. The dialogical praxis developed by Paulo Freire (1989a, 1989b, 1985; Freire and Macedo, 1987) does this impressively. It shares the value base we have described at the same time that its theory of practice is both phenomenological and Marxist. Freire is committed to raising a worker's and a client's consciousness as Subjects meeting in the world and would not be opposed, we believe, to having this done in both the Freudian and Marxist senses (Aronowitz, 1993):

The dialogical theory of action does not involve a Subject, who dominates by virtue of conquest, and a dominated object. Instead there are Subjects who meet to name the world in order

> to transform it. . . . Cooperation leads dialogical Subjects to focus their attention on the reality which mediates them which—posed as a problem—challenges them. (Freire, 1989a, pp. 167-168)

The starting point to identify, explore, analyze, understand, and engage the contradictions among values, theory, and practice is the clinical encounter. Generally, the worker must deal with his or her own contradictions before work on the contradictions in the agency, profession, or political economy takes place. Exploration at the worker level will, however, often illuminate issues at the level of the agency, profession, and so on, which will require engagement if contradictions in clinical work are to be understood.

The concept of contradictions is central to bridging the gap between clinical work and social action. By contradictions, we mean the inconsistencies, discrepancies, antagonisms, or lack of truth (Guralnick, 1970) between what workers, agencies, professions, and social institutions profess and the actions in which they actually engage. Contradictions occur at different levels and their content and form will vary. Yet, political, economic, and emotional interests are at play that prevent workers and organizations from examining, engaging, and attempting to resolve contradictions.

For example, agencies often force students and workers to deal with client fees at the beginning of a therapeutic session. This policy contradicts both the values of client self-determination and psychodynamic formulations that suggest that one ought to allow a client to begin a session. The above example also illuminates the contradictions faced by a social service agency, which is under market-driven financial pressures despite its commitment to serve clients regardless of their ability to pay. Issues related to third-party payers, the economics of managed care, and a host of other social justice issues are also involved.

These contradictions also precipitate psychological effects. Clients may react defensively or angrily at the worker when the worker asks for fee payment. The worker may become defensive and angry at the agency and project that anger on the client in the form of victim blaming. Each of these issues—profits versus people, money versus service, social control versus self-determination—and their psychological effects has a potential for clinical work and social action. Naming and addressing contradictions is a powerful force for change.

Teaching from a Freirian perspective in a university-based human services program represents another contradiction (Leonard, 1993). In the university, a Freirian approach invariably will produce tensions between "normal" pedagogy that imparts content and a Freirian pedagogy that poses content through a dialogical praxis. This approach focuses on problem posing rather than lecturing; between the expectations of the professor role on the part of both the school and the students, and the professor as a participant in a process of dialogical learning. For Freire, there is a tension between meeting in the world as equal Subjects and the expectation that the professor assign grades and otherwise objectify the work of students.

These contradictions remove the teacher from the relative comfort and safety of a familiar role and place the students in a similarly unfamiliar position. Attempts to manage and/or reactions to the tensions created by this new pedagogy, while remaining within the institution, vary widely. For some students, the inconsistencies between university ideology and Freirian practice are often a source of great anxiety and/or anger. For other students, it is an exciting opportunity to take control of their learning. Faculty who choose to move in this direction must be prepared to give up their privileged position and the power that comes with it.

The practice model we propose will challenge the silence and acceptance of the current splits between values, theory, and practice and forthrightly identify and engage—if not always resolve—the resulting contradictions. This model simultaneously addresses the unique intrapsychic dynamics and processes of the individual and the unique contents, dynamics, and processes of the social world that the individual has internalized and is living in. To uncover these dimensions will require an ongoing dialogical praxis that is capable of examining the motives and meanings embedded in the social actions (Freund, 1969) of different actors in the clinical encounter. It will also require a praxis that does not shrink from the implications for social action that emerge from the examination of the contradictions in clinical work.

It is our view that political and economic justice issues, though not always apparent on the surface, are embedded in every clinical encounter. At times they are illuminated through an examination of unconscious material such as dreams and transference manifestations (Fanon, 1967; Lieberman, 1988). This is part of a clinician's work. Similarly, we believe that all work on political and economic justice issues has embedded within it psychological components that need to be addressed.

We can think of no better way to end this introduction and begin the process of exploring and building a practice to bridge the false dichotomy between clinical work and social action than to relate a piece of dialogue from a discussion between Paulo Freire and a group of human service workers and faculty. When asked how it is possible to do progressive work in the context of an oppressive and antagonistic structure, he responded with a story. He pointed out that whether one is working in an agency or in a university or is a revolutionary in the mountains, one always has a foot in each of two worlds. "That," he remarked, "is why I walk so funny."

A central question of this book is: What can be done within the contradictions that are bound to exist as we struggle to find a way to work authentically? We recognize that this book is a beginning attempt to walk down "a road less traveled." But, as Paulo Freire and Myles Horton, activist and educator, point out (Horton and Freire, 1990): "We make the road by walking." The story we related above will, we hope, explain why it is that we walk with funny gaits and often stumble.

OUTLINE OF THE BOOK

Chapter 2—Values

Social welfare work is value based. Theory may be used to understand how a client and worker may move from point A to point B, but it is values that ought to determine which point B a worker and client agree to move toward.

Chapter 2 identifies and examines in detail the three values that guide our selection and utilization of theory and are key to the practice model that we will develop and use. The tensions and conflicts that exist within and between values as well as the practice implications our values have in relation to the political economy, profession, agency, and clinical work will be addressed.

As noted, the central values we hold are:

- self-determination of communities, groups, families, and individuals;
- economic and political justice; and
- a belief and commitment to dialogical praxis (Freire, 1989a).

Chapters 3 to 6—Theory

Chapter 3 begins by introducing the necessity, usefulness, meanings, and practical implications of having a relatively integrated set of theories that are in sync with the three values explored in Chapter 2. The chapter then moves on to a discussion of phenomenological theory and methods. The chapter ends with a detailed case example that illustrates the usefulness of phenomenological theory and methods.

Chapter 4 focuses on selected aspects of Freudian and neo-Freudian psychology. It explores the usefulness of analyzing and understanding an individual's unconscious structures and processes and how the content of the unconscious is related to larger social structures.

Chapter 5 describes and analyzes some of the major theories developed in sociology that led up to the development of symbolic interaction theory. At the end of the chapter, symbolic interaction theory is used to develop and extend an analysis of Hispanic lesbian clients first developed in a paper by DeMonteflores (1981).

Chapter 6 is devoted to critical theory. Particular attention will be devoted to the roots of critical theorists and their attempt to integrate the work of Marx and Freud. At the end of the chapter, we will briefly and critically explore the development and usefulness of postmodern theory.

The theories presented in Chapters 3 to 6 are purposefully meant to be overlapping and complementary. The ways these theories can be used to check, balance, and reinforce one another will be demonstrated. In addition, numerous examples of their application to practice and their connection to the work of Paulo Freire will be presented.

Chapter 7—Contradictions

Chapter 7 is devoted to the concept of contradictions. Contradictions will be explored at the level of the worker, the agency, the profession, social work education, and the political economy.

Chapter 8—Work with the Homeless

Chapter 8 presents a detailed case example of work with a group of homeless people, carried out by one of the authors. The work was informed by our values, selected parts of our theory base and, most important, the practice and pedagogy developed by Paulo Freire.

Chapters 9 to 14—Teaching and Case Examples

Chapters 9 to 14 describe in detail the issues and techniques related to teaching this model of practice in a university setting. We will draw heavily on our experience during the past seven years of teaching our course as well as our experience running professional workshops and institutes.

Chapter 9 introduces our teaching and presents the first day of one of our classes. It includes a discussion of the ways students can expect teaching and learning to be different in a class using our model and how a student's learning objectives can be usefully problematized (Freire, 1985).

Chapter 10 focuses on a case discussion related to the contradictions, practice issues, and conflicts a student experienced in her work with a gay man who was also a practicing Christian.

Chapter 11 introduces the use of codifications and a discussion of the codifications developed by students in our class. These codifications were representations of their experiences in their field internships and in summer classes at Smith.

Chapters 12 and 13 examine the work described in a process recording of an African-American student worker with an African-American client. Included in these chapters are clinical and social action issues related to starting a session, power, community violence, supervision, agency work, and community organizing.

Chapter 14 explores the three-part written assignment we ask students to do over the course of the semester and the dialogical process that is created.

The epilogue returns both philosophically and pragmatically to the contradictions workers will experience if they hope to practice in a progressive way in the United States during the twenty-first century. We will address the dilemmas workers are likely to face as they attempt to introduce this model into their work with clients in the context of current and future agency practice.

Chapter 2

Values

It all begins with values. Social work is a value-based profession. Social workers make this statement with pride. We have values and we make those values the basis of our clinical work, advocacy, and public policy agenda. We choose to work with people who are oppressed—people no other profession embraces—because of these values.

Social work's values have been the subject of considerable discussion and scholarly effort over the years:

> The profession of social work historically has been committed to enhancing the welfare of people who encounter problems related to poverty, mental health, health care, employment, shelter and housing, abuse, aging, childhood, hunger, and so on. As the profession has evolved, it has continually stressed the need to attend both to the needs of individual clients, and to the ways that the community and society respond to those needs. Thus, there has always been a simultaneous concern in social work for individual well-being and the environmental factors that affect it. (Reamer, 1995, pp. 893-894)

Social work's value base is codified in the *NASW Code of Ethics,* last revised in 1997. "The sections of the current code set forth principles related to the social worker's general conduct and comportment and ethical responsibilities to clients, colleagues, employing organizations, the social work profession and society" (Reamer, 1995, p. 896). Although other organizations, notably the National Association of Black Social Workers and the Society of Clinical Social Work Psychotherapists, have created their own codes, it is NASW's that serves as the most widely recognized articulation of the profession's values.

The fact that social work is a value-based profession is also used to belittle the field. Values, according to that perspective, should be secondary to "scientific rigor" in the selection of theories we use to guide our practice or of the policies we choose to promote. Social workers are accused of being led by their hearts instead of their heads and, therefore, advancing theories and practice approaches not because they work but because they "feel right." That would be a telling criticism if all theory and practice were not also value driven.

> One cannot be a social worker and be like the educator who's a coldly neutral technician. To keep our options secret, to conceal them in the cobwebs of technique, or to disguise them by claiming neutrality does not constitute neutrality; quite the contrary, it helps maintain the status quo. (Freire, 1985, p. 39)

We note Freire's comment on professional neutrality to underscore our own commitment to be explicit about our values, to make clear what we believe and how what we believe is related to the selection of our theory base and practice goals and methods. Our values challenge the status quo. For this reason, we utilize theories that are consistent with those values, theories that help us to understand and deal with conflict, and theories that will inform a practice that challenges oppressive aspects of the status quo.

As we noted in Chapter 1, the central values we propose to direct and guide practice are:

- self-determination of communities, groups, families, and individuals;
- economic and political justice; and
- a belief in and commitment to dialogical praxis. (Freire, 1989a, 1985)

In this chapter, we will discuss these values, show how they relate to theory and practice, how they relate to each other, and how we deal with the conflicts that, at times, exist among them.

SELF-DETERMINATION

The idea of self-determination implies knowledge of one's world as well as the means to act on that world (Freire, 1989a). Communal interests, in our view, take priority over those of the individual. Therefore, self-determination begins with the community and not with individuals, as it is usually formulated. The reason for this "new" formulation is that individual interests may be selfish and self-serving and often conflict with the interests of the community. Marx noted "the seemingly complete independence of the individual, who mistakes for personal freedom the unrestrained control of his alienated vital elements . . . is no longer checked by ties to the community" (quoted in Bloch, 1966, p. 222). The right to individual property can limit the rights of other individuals and the community as a whole (Bloch, 1966). Our value holds that the rights of the community of citizens override the property rights of individual men or women.

Our view of communal interest is grounded in an analysis of oppression which suggests that oppression at the individual level is generally a manifestation of the oppression of the group of which the individual is a member. For example, while discrimination against women is variously described as resulting from patriarchy (Miller, 1992) or capitalism (Abramovitz, 1988), both theorists agree that the oppression of women serves the interests of a ruling elite whose interests are not communal. In this context, it is not enough that an individual woman has the opportunity to rise to become part of the elite. For us, what is critical is that the community of women should no longer be oppressed. Similarly, we are committed to the communal liberation of people of color, the poor, people with disabilities, gays and lesbians—that is, all people who suffer institutional oppression. Further, we challenge the sectarian view of self-determination in which groups are encouraged to think and act only in terms of the group's self-interest rather than as part of the larger class of oppressed people.

Self-determination, we believe, is liberating and, for us, it is a strongly held value. In its essence, self-determination speaks to the right of communities, groups, families, and individuals to make, or at least be involved in, decisions that affect their lives. This principle provides a clear set of directions to a worker as to how he or she conducts an interview. It demands that a social worker understand and act on the needs and interests of a family in the family's terms. In a like manner, self-determination places social workers on the side of communities that are being acted upon by outside social institutional forces over which they have little control, but which decisively affect the members of that community. This does not hold for communities that are out to oppress others because that would violate our commitment to economic and political justice.

The social work literature on self-determination tends to focus on the individual. Questions related to the tension between client self-determination and the responsibility of the social worker to "protect" the client from foolish or dangerous choices is a frequent theme. The concern that some clients—the developmentally disabled, those with mental illness diagnoses, those in weakened physical states, the too-young—may be unable to exercise "true" self-determination because of these conditions is used as a justification for weakening this core principle of social welfare practice. Although there certainly are instances in which a community, group, family, or individual client may be unable to articulate a clear statement of their wishes, we argue for a skeptical stance in regard to situations of that sort. The tendency toward paternalism—toward treating a client as an Object rather than a Subject—is strongly embedded in the professional role and must be resisted through a process of dialogue with the client and honest reflection on the part of the worker. We would suggest that the tendency toward paternalism in social service agencies is at least partly a reflection of the unwillingness of social workers and their agencies to give up or share some of their power with clients. True dialogue with clients implies a sharing of power.

The clinical encounter is the starting point for self-determination to be realized. The client determines what will happen in the session by identifying the issues to be discussed, and by choosing whether to accept or reject the worker's observations, suggestions, or interpretations. At the most basic level, the client exercises choice as to whether to return for subsequent sessions. Too frequently, we know that the client does not return (Baekeland and Lundwall, 1975). We may, as a consequence, label the client resistant or "hard to reach," rather than seeing the issue in the worker or the agency.

But, self-determination has another side. The very notion is based in the individualistic ideology of capitalism. "I can do what I want; it's my life." "No one can tell me what to do; this is a free country." These are typical expressions of that ideology. And, from one perspective, they are compelling and appealing. No one wants to be told what to do. Nor is it common in our individually focused capitalist society for people to make their own wishes and desires secondary to a consideration of the public good. A drive along any road, littered with trash thrown from passing cars, offers disturbing testimony to the power of that belief.

Capitalist ideology, at its essence, promotes the kinds of social irresponsibility reflected in the previous example. In its exaltation of individual self-interest, there is no rational reason why motorists should foul their own cars when the mess can be transferred to property owned by all of us collectively or to another individual. American culture has become increasingly willing to permit individuals and corporations to act on their own self-interest and to pass on the cost of the consequences to all of us. We see utility companies contaminating rivers with toxic waste and the tobacco industry disregarding the public's health. Corporations make decisions to relocate factories to low-wage developing countries while destroying the economic and social fabric of communities in this country. The mania to cut taxes for the rich has disrupted and destroyed lives by withdrawing funds needed to provide public benefits. There has been an overall willingness to allow corporations to dominate public life. This is permitted so long as basic needs are met, and more radical desires are diverted through the process of repressive desublimation (Marcuse, 1966).

This country saw its origins in the desire of people to live their lives freely, throwing off the despotic demands of a monarch—the personification of the state who could abridge individual and collective liberties and confiscate individual and collective property. American ideas of liberty and property are grounded in individualism. It is not surprising, therefore, that the United States has developed a political ethos based on suspicion of a powerful state. Our entire system of government is based on checks and balances to prevent any one branch of government from becoming too influential. We are, it is clear, more willing to endure governmental gridlock than to permit an activist government to institute wide-ranging policies that could infringe on personal liberty or property rights.

Our history, of course, is more complex than the dominant discourse we've described. Although individual freedom and property rights were of major importance to the colonists and to subsequent settlers, those freedoms were not extended to the Native peoples already living here, nor to Africans brought here as property, nor to the Chinese whose labor made much of the Western expansion possible (Weaver, 1998). Women were not permitted to own property, vote, or be accorded the full privileges of citizenship for nearly a century and a half after the signing of the Declaration of Independence (Davis, 1983; Abramovitz, 1988). There are privileged classes whose individual freedom and personal property are to be respected and others whose individuality is not bound to be honored.

It is the desire to operate as a free agent, unaccountable to a powerful state, that makes it so difficult to advance collective solutions to public issues of social structure because they are viewed as individual troubles, that is, a private matter (Mills, 1961). To the extent that the problems we see people bringing to human service organizations are defined as "individual," as resulting from some dysfunction in the person seeking services, then the ability to mobilize a collective response to them is at odds with popular consciousness. Social work has a responsibility to "swim against the current" in that context. It must assert a public responsibility and advocate collective solutions to issues having their origins in political and economic institutions as opposed to the personal troubles of individuals. "An issue, in fact, often involves what Marxists call 'contradictions' or 'antagonisms'" (Mills, 1961, p. 9). The current issue of welfare reform is one example of how a social problem created and sustained by political and economic institutions is being defined as a personal trouble, as demonstrated in the Personal Responsibility and Work Opportunity Reconciliation Act of 1996. "Both the correct statement of the problem and the range of possible solutions requires us to consider the economic and political institutions of society, and not merely the personal situations and character of a scatter of individuals" (Mills, 1961, p. 9). A collective solution to this issue would be such things as universal child care allowances, a guaranteed annual wage above the poverty level and living-wage jobs, day care, adequate low cost housing, and so forth. The meeting of these human necessities would then allow for people to be truly self-determining.

Self-determination, then, is laden with contradictory impulses and influences. At its best, it is a value that obligates us to help clients come to an understanding of their world and provide a means for acting on it. Clients, it should be noted, can be individuals or families, groups, or communities. While clinical work has traditionally been seen as work with individuals and families, in our framework it embraces a much larger view of the people with whom we are engaged. A large part of our work will still be done with individuals or small groups, but our conception of the client leaves room to have a broader vision. Whenever possible, opportunities should be sought that bring individuals, families, and groups together, particularly when the issues they are dealing with affect them collectively as well as personally.

In practice, this means that we raise questions that not only clarify what clients are saying but that invite them to think more deeply about the forces that have brought them to the situation they are in. "The social worker who opts for change strives to unveil reality" (Freire, 1985, p. 40), and does this through dialogue with the client. Clinical dialogue is joined with collective action to change the world through the process of dialogical praxis.

ECONOMIC AND POLITICAL JUSTICE

There are many definitions of the terms economic and political justice—some academic, some rhetorical, all attempting to provide some words for what most people seem to understand intuitively, if not consistently. One statement that captures the spirit of economic and political justice and defines it in eloquent and behavioral terms was made by American socialist leader Eugene Victor Debs. He said: "While there is a lower class, I am in it. While there is a criminal element, I am of it. While there is a soul in jail, I am not free" (Debs, 1966, p. 110). Debs' statement captures the stance we take in regard to economic and political justice: it is an identification with the lives and struggles of people who are oppressed.

In a capitalist society, most conceptions of justice are individual. People are entitled to live their lives unencumbered by restrictions on their freedom to act according to their own needs and desires. Freedom, according to this framework, is to be limited only in the most compelling of circumstances, such as the protection of the life or property of another person. At the end of the twentieth century, even these restrictions are the subject of spirited debate. Individuals who wish to develop land, for example, are increasingly presumed to be able to do so even if their plans will adversely affect the health and safety or property rights of others.

As we have said, we propose an alternative vision, one that is grounded in collective economic and political justice. In this context, our vision of economic and political justice stands in opposition to the individualistic view of self-determination. We would prefer to have decisions which have often been viewed as "private" be subject to a test that questions and assesses the impact of those decisions on the larger collective—society, community, group, and family. A corporation, for example, which has received public benefits, such as tax incentives, would not be permitted to close a plant if it would devastate a local community. In an economic and political justice-centered framework, the social cost of unemployment would be weighed against the presumed right of an individual company to act in its narrow self-interest.

In the case of Mary, whom we met in Chapter 1, the social cost of unemployment comes into her home. She comes to the session with her worker and describes her boyfriend Larry's display of a gun as part of his erratic behavior following the loss of his job at the local factory. The factory was laying people off, and his job ended, as did his opportunity to attend college.

A commitment to economic and political justice requires us to work with Mary to ensure that her safety is provided for. That is the first priority because of the potential for violence against her. We would, however, want to examine what we might do for her boyfriend in the face of his involuntary unemployment. In an era of downsizing, Mary's situation is being played out in many homes throughout the community. Unemployment often leads to domestic violence, substance abuse, and mental illness.

Holding a job is equated with masculinity in a society that social-izes men to be breadwinners. This socialization also has, at least implicitly, given men permission to turn their felt powerlessness in the larger world into dominating behavior in their intimate relation-ships (Carlson, 1977; Davis, 1987; Pease, 1997). The phenomena of displacement and/or "identification with the oppressor" (Sachs, 1991) are very likely at play here—an analytic frame that is more consistent with our values than labeling Larry's behavior as socio-pathic or seeing him as someone either intrinsically violent or un-worthy of support. Another issue is easy access to guns—a political issue that is often implicated in domestic violence situations that turn deadly. Informed by our values, a worker would want to bring Larry, together with his former co-workers at the factory and devel-op a political response to the layoffs. This would direct their aggres-sion and anger productively back where it belongs, at the corpora-tion that laid them off.

If we are to act on our commitment to political and economic justice, what are we then to do? First, we work with Mary to develop a plan for her safety. In the conversation between Mary and the worker, Mary described her discussion with a police detective. There she got some clarity about what was possible within the law and what the very real limitations were. The law offers only limited protection to women fearing domestic violence. Our response would be to work with Mary, women like her, and progressive men to provide more services, including legal services, to abused and threat-ened women in the community. Ideally, this would eventually in-clude Larry and his co-workers.

Our concern for political and economic justice would have us attempt to reform the law. We would seek more creative and pro-active responses from the police to help women in Mary's situation. Law reform offers an opportunity for work at the community level and for thinking about Mary's concerns about her own safety as a larger political issue.

Part of the work, however, is still individual. A key element in any community intervention would be to work with Mary to identi-fy policies that would be helpful to her. We would need to identify the supports she would need to move this issue from a purely personal trouble to a broader political and economic framework. In this context, supports include interpersonal work to allow her to feel her strength sufficiently to raise the issue in larger arenas. Other supports would be needed from the community to address her concerns in a substantive manner. Having done that, the second part of our intervention would be community organizing.

The relationship between unemployment, domestic violence, and easy access to guns leads us to look for approaches that provide safety for Mary. After ensuring Mary's safety, we then need to identify ways to address the social issue of domestic violence. We do this by building a coalition of people in the community who have an interest in this problem. This coalition would be most effective if it embraced a wide range of worldviews but agreed on a common objective (Alexander, 1991; Kahn, 1991).

In this situation, we might be looking for traditional allies: women's organizations, domestic violence prevention programs, and social service organizations. In addition, we also want to explore the interest of law enforcement agencies such as the police, the district attorney's office, and the courts. We would seek support from Larry's union, local churches, and local civic and business groups. The issue of domestic violence might help the community build support for an effort to push the corporation to consider the negative impacts of their economic decisions. This initial exploration of coalition partners suggests the potential for turning Mary's issue into part of a larger campaign for economic and political justice.

Similarly, we need to ask how we can engage Larry and the other men in his community who face corporate downsizing. To do that it would be important to meet with Larry individually and in a group of his peers to look at how gender influences his way of experiencing, understanding, and expressing his anger. We do know that Larry's rage and confusion are closely related to the actions of an employer acting in its own interest. That employer feels little sense of accountability to the community that has provided its workforce. Rather than taking out his rage on Mary, he might be helped to direct that anger at a more deserving target—the corporation. Working with Larry in this way can increase the safety of Mary and other women in the community.

Dealing with economic issues would mean meeting with Larry and his co-workers in their union hall, at the local bowling alley, the local bar, and so on. Engaging Larry and his friends on their turf would equalize the power between them and the worker and create a Subject to Subject relationship (Burghardt, 1982; Freire, 1989a). This is in contrast to expecting Larry and his friends to come to the agency where they might well feel stigmatized, alienated, and/or pathologized.

It is clear that Larry cannot act alone if he is to have any chance at success. Working with other men and women in the community to develop a collective understanding of their situation is a place to start. Supporting unionization efforts—or an existing union—would be helpful. Former co-workers and their allies will need to be brought together to put pressure on elected officials to engage in strategies to force the factory owners either to maintain their investment in the community or to provide meaningful economic reparations. The critical element is to help local workers avoid reacting to their situation as if they were personally at fault. This is a natural reaction in an individualistically oriented society.

DIALOGICAL PRAXIS

A belief in dialogical praxis is the third value that informs our work. Dialogical praxis is a *process of action and reflection between two Subjects* (people who accord each other equal worth) *who meet to examine and transform their world*. Because this concept is fairly complex, it will be useful to examine the elements of the definition of dialogical praxis and clarify the values embedded within it.

Dialogical praxis is first a process, an ongoing, interactive relationship. The process includes a commitment to the relationship. We are prepared to keep on talking, to work through whatever issues arise within the relationship or emerge from it. Process takes place over time, thus permitting a developing trust, depth, and communion (Freire, 1989a) between the participants.

Praxis is action and reflection, which means that you say or do something, get a response, reflect on it, say something else, listen, reflect on it, and so on. The critical idea here is that neither reflective thinking nor doing, by itself, is enough. Reflective thinking, in this context, means more than just casual thought—it involves a deep introspection that can be political and sometimes painful in its revelations (Freire, 1989a). Acting, in the clinical sense, often means saying something, offering a response to the client's statement with the goal of moving the process along.

In our approach, the worker's response should reflect self-determination and economic and political justice. Any response on the part of the worker represents a decision, a choice from among a multitude of options. The choice of what element of a client's statement to respond to should flow from reflective thought about the options available. Concern is often expressed that choosing a response based on a personal value is an imposition of the worker's "agenda" on the clinical encounter. We respond to this concern in two ways: first, our commitment to self-determination would be violated were we to attempt to coerce the client's response—we would be acting in contradiction to our values. Second, we recognize and support clients' power to make their own choices about the direction of the work they do with us. We do not, however, pretend a neutrality that does not exist (Freire, 1985).

A Subject-to-Subject relationship is one in which each party recognizes the worth of the other. Seeing the client as an objectified other—as "The Client," for example—while assuming a role as the "The Expert" or "The Professional" would be a violation of the commitment to dialogical praxis. This is particularly difficult in the increasingly hierarchical agency settings in which workers are employed in a system dominated by managed care. A worker's role frequently is to "fix" the clients or to relieve their distress sufficiently that they will no longer seek service. A person does not "fix" an equal, so the commitment to a Subject-to-Subject relationship requires great attention (much reflection) lest the worker fall into an "expert" position to meet the needs of the employer.

The purpose of dialogical praxis is to provide an opportunity for two equals to meet to examine and transform their world. Examination of the world has its roots in reflection and action. The reflection engaged in by client and worker is directed to an increased understanding of the different forces that affect their lives. Sometimes these forces are internal, sometimes external. But these forces are present in and affect the clinical setting.

In the example we are using in this chapter, we would explore the limits of the ability of the police to ensure Mary's safety if Larry should attempt to harm her. We would question who benefits from the inadequacy of policies related to domestic violence. We would also ask how Larry might direct his anger at the employer who has thwarted his ambitions rather than at Mary. Exploring the client's world includes inquiry into the larger forces that affect them. In addition, the worker might reflect on her role as a woman in a social welfare agency that may also be affected by corporate downsizing.

Dialogical praxis can, and often must, help us to reconcile tensions between our commitment to political and economic justice and our commitment to self-determination. It can, for example, allow us to explore a client's racism or sexism or heterosexism in terms of the forces at play—sociopolitical and psychological—in the client's presentation of self. Concepts such as "identification with the aggressor" and "internalized oppression" could be explored in this context. It also requires us to look at those elements in our own reactions to the client's world.

Action after reflection—reflection provides a vehicle for the worker to assess the extent to which an intervention contradicts his or her values or is consistent with them. The ideal is to reflect, recognize, and act on contradictions between one's values and one's practice. For example, some of our students were decidedly unsympathetic to Larry, were not interested in his issues or needs, and would easily have seen him thrown in jail or castrated before feeling any empathy for the economic and political issues that affected his life. Likewise, the agency's expectations, the worker's countertransference, and/or society's attitude toward domestic violence could all leave the blame for this situation with Larry as an individual. Blaming Larry would contradict our values of political and economic justice for workers and self-determination for Larry. We would not deny Larry's responsibility for his behavior but rather acknowledge that the forces that led to it must also be addressed.

Similarly, the race, gender, or sexual orientation of a client can create institutional forces that will increase the likelihood of workers taking actions that will place them in contradiction with their values. For example, the institutional racism, classism, sexism, or homophobia of an agency could influence the pathologizing or devaluing of clients.

If we return to Mary and Larry, we can see how this might work in the kinds of complex situations workers frequently confront. Justice demands that we oppose domestic violence, while self-determination permits clients their own beliefs. A commitment to reflection and action provides the means for helping the worker deal with a seemingly intractable contradiction—how to avoid either giving support through silence to unjust beliefs or actions, or denying the client the right to freely express those beliefs.

In the situation we have explored in this chapter, it is clear that Mary is concerned for her physical safety as well as for Larry's well-being. She believes, probably with some basis, that Larry really would not harm her and that he is in a great deal of pain and turmoil. Larry, were he to be seen by the worker, might acknowledge that his behavior was wrong. He might also minimize the legitimacy of Mary's frightened reaction. In this case, a worker would need to engage Larry in a way that would facilitate his ability to deeply reflect on the meanings attached to his handgun.

A worker seeing Mary and Larry would have to find a way to talk about supporting each of them without downplaying each of their understandings of their struggles.

Chapter 3

Introduction to Theory
and Phenomenology

[I]f radicals wish to change their world, they must surely expect to do so only against the resistance of some and with the help of others. Yet those whom they oppose, as well as those with whom they wish to ally themselves, will in fact often be guided by certain theories. Without self-conscious theory, radicals will be unable to understand, let alone change, either their enemies or their friends. Radicals who believe that they can separate the task of developing theory from that of changing society are not in fact acting without a theory, but with one that is tacit and therefore unexaminable and uncorrectable.

Alvin W. Gouldner
The Coming Crisis of Western Sociology, p. 5

A central value of this work is our belief and commitment to dialogical praxis, the process of action and reflection between two Subjects who meet to talk about, examine, understand, and transform their world. For us, it is in the world of social welfare agencies in the context of the larger society that subjects, that is, human service workers and communities, groups, families, and individuals, meet and have the opportunity to engage in dialogical praxis. This world is the subject of our investigation and our praxis. For the value of dialogical praxis to be operationalized, we need a set of theories that provide both the knowledge and the methodologies to identify and reflect on the contextual world of human service workers and the people they engage in their work. The theoretical examination and understanding of the world of these relationships will then lead to the development of plans that can operationalize our other central values, that is, collective self-determined social actions that promote economic and political justice.

As a part of our praxis, we expect the knowledge and methodologies embedded in the theories selected to be examined. They cannot be split off or be in contradiction to our values or our practice. They cannot be, as Cooper (1977, p. 363) suggested of most social work writing, a "Sears Roebuck listing of knowledge" that has created a fragmented situation in which social workers display rather than integrate knowledge for use (Bartlett, 1970). Indeed, if our theory and the practice model it informs contradict our values, then the theory and model will need to be modified or changed. In this way, clarity, consistency, and authenticity in our praxis and our work can be maintained. Workers and clients, as well as politicians, administrators, and policymakers at all levels may choose to share, disagree with, or critique our values. This dialogue will reveal potential allies, adversaries, and those with whom further dialogue could be productive.

We recognize that no theory, including the selected theories we use, is value free. Theoretical ideas most often reflect dominant and prevailing social, economic, and political interests. In addition, theories also reflect the idiosyncratic feelings, affective states, sentiments (Gouldner, 1970), and psychological character of individual theorists and the people, including workers, who use theory.

The selected theories we use are consciously chosen to inform and guide actions that will lead to the attainment of our values. It is essential and decisive whether a critique of our theory and methods reveals contradictions with our values. When a critique reveals contradictions between values, theory, and methods, it will be a signal that the theory and/or methods require change. Values are not open to question. They are the fixed point against which contradictions can be examined.

The theories selected are purposefully overlapping and complementary. They check, balance, and reinforce one another. Each, in different ways, promotes reflection and consciousness raising and has the potential to reveal contradictions and conflicts that may exist between theories, between theory and practice, and between theory, practice, and our value commitments. For example, Freud's theory of unconscious processes could help explain the contradictions and examine the hidden meanings of a worker who voices a value about engaging an agency's oppressive actions but fails to do so. In this example, the contradiction could reflect unconscious motives related to the workers' anxiety about losing his or her job or negative countertransference issues related to the people he or she works with, such as unconscious prejudices related to a client's race, class, gender, sexual orientation, and so on.

On the other hand, symbolic interaction theory's understanding of how the contents of a culture are internalized (Mead, 1934) and critical theory's emphasis on examining social institutions when trying to understand a social problem (Findlay, 1978) are useful in examining some aspects of biological determinism in Freudian theory. For example, they would help explain Freud's ideas related to gender issues, for example, men's purported rationality and women's purported emotionality. Freud's socialization in patriarchal Viennese culture is clearly evident in the part of his theory that speaks to the emotional and task roles women and men are expected to play (Mead, 1934). In addition, critical theory would allow us to observe and critique the ways that this part of Freud's theory has been used and abused to maintain gender inequality in social institutions. These reflective critiques could then inform the next action part of our praxis. Specifically, the idea that particular groups of, or individual, women or men are more emotional or more intellectual at a particular moment, on a particular day, or in general would never negate the value of their remaining in dialogue and participating in decision making. We would necessarily see their emotional and intellectual contributions as essential to the dialogue. The world could then be understood deeply, both emotionally and intellectually. This understanding could then lead to actions that attempt to eliminate or reduce gender inequality in social institutions, including human service agencies.

With this introduction to the role of theory, we will now more deeply enter phenomenological theory and explore how it can serve our praxis. No attempt will be made to present all of phenomenological theory or all of the other theories we have chosen. This would be impossible given the space available and the extensive writings of Freud, Marx, Mead, Husserl, and Freire, and so on, let alone those who have interpreted and extended them. Our hope is to open selected aspects of a theory that can guide and inform a worker's praxis in a way that keeps faith with our values. Case material will be presented to illustrate, explore, explain, and demonstrate the value of the central theoretical ideas and concepts that we have chosen.

PHENOMENOLOGY, THE CRITICAL INCIDENT TECHNIQUE, PROCESS RECORDING, AND PROBLEMATIZING THE WORLD

Phenomenological theory and methods have influenced Paulo Freire's (1989a) work, have shaped and been shaped by psychoanalytic theory and methods (Ricoeur, 1970), have influenced critical theory (Horkheimer, 1937; Roderick, 1986), and have paralleled some aspects of symbolic interaction theory (Berger and Luckman, 1966; Luckman, 1978). It is essential to our praxis that phenomenology moves us, in Husserl's words, to *"dich an sich,"* i.e., to *the thing itself.* For human service workers doing clinical work, the thing itself is the clinical encounter. The clinical encounter includes those structures and processes, both psychological and sociological, that interact constantly between workers and the people they serve in social institutional contexts.

What follows are methods that we have found useful to identify the world of clinical work. These methods are based in a set of phenomenological ideas that promote reflection on the clinical process, an essential ingredient in our praxis.

The use of Flanagan's (1954) critical incident technique and a worker's process recordings (essentially a series of critical incidents) are two major ways to begin to locate the world, *the thing itself,* of clinical social work. Both critical incidents and process recordings identify the world to be reflected upon:

> By an incident is meant any observable human activity that is sufficiently complete in itself to permit inferences and predictions to be made about the person performing the act. To be critical, an incident must occur in a situation where the purpose or intent of the act seems fairly clear to the observer and where its consequences are sufficiently definite to leave little doubt concerning its effects. (Flanagan, 1954, p. 327)

This technique has proven successful in gathering rich and clear descriptions of a worker's practice. Practice descriptions have come from a variety of personnel, including social welfare workers. Flanagan observed that since its development, the critical incident technique had gained wide use by a large number of researchers in areas ranging from job training to counseling and psychotherapy.

How does phenomenology inform reflection on the world of clinical encounters that have been identified by the critical incident technique? Natanson suggests that:

> Phenomenology begins with the strangeness of experience. . . . It involves a radical stance, a remarkable way of looking at things. That experience cannot be taken straightforwardly, that it is to-be-understood, introduces a mode of reversal into the ordinary and unreflective acceptance of the mundane course of affairs: a philosophical turn of mind signifies a shifting of perspective from simple placement in the world to wonder about it aslant. (1967, pp. 182, 184)

This follows the social phenomenologist Alfred Schutz's ideas about people's *taken-for-granted world*.

> The taken-for-granted is always that particular level of experience which presents itself as not in need of further analysis. Whether a level of experience is thus taken for granted depends on the pragmatic interest of the reflective glance which is directed upon it and thereby upon the particular Here and Now from which that glance is operating. To say that some content of consciousness is thus taken for granted still leaves it open as to whether any kind of existence or reality is credited to that content, i.e., whether it is given in acts of positional or neutral consciousness. Nevertheless, a change of attention can transform something that is taken for granted into something problematic. (Schutz, 1967, p. 74)

This mode of inquiry is not totally new to human service workers and to social workers in particular. Workers by themselves or with their supervisors have always reflected on their work. The intensity and rigor of phenomenology, however, does add a deeper dimension to what has been an important, but too often prematurely dropped, element of inquiry into the complexity of meanings. "Serious study," to quote Paulo Freire (1985), "requires not merely critical penetration into . . . basic content but also penetration into an acute sensibility, a permanent intellectual disquiet, a predisposition to investigation" (p. 3). Phenomenology can foster, indeed requires, this disquiet. The disquiet is essential when reflecting on the economics and politics embedded in critical incidents. In this mode of inquiry, workers and others reflecting on a worker's interventions are encouraged to see more and explain contradictions and gaps in the data about actions that have been observed (Glaser and Strauss, 1967).

In addition, Natanson (1967) would require that the phenomenon to be analyzed must be approached from a presuppositional point of view, a view which embodies "a primordial strangeness":

> The situation of primordial strangeness must be attended to on its own, examined in its givenness, and expressed in a language which is finely sensitive to the meaning it seeks to articulate. The "language of reality" does more than report; it reconstructs, and it does so through a rhetoric which is resonant with its object. (Natanson, 1967, p. 188)

For phenomenologists, it is not the causal explanation of a phenomenon that is of greatest interest. More impressive is the rigorous examination of the essential elements related to a phenomenon and the context in which the phenomenon is lodged. Our interest is in the complexity and configurations of meanings, motivations, and contexts that surround and are embedded in the slice of the world that is being investigated. In Freire's words, the meaning of that part of the world that is problematized is essential.

> Problematization is the antithesis of "problem solving." In problem solving, an expert takes distance from reality and reduces it to dimensions which are amenable to treatment as though they were mere difficulties to be solved. To "problematize" is to engage a group in the task of codifying reality into symbols which can generate critical consciousness and empower them to alter their relations with nature and oppressive social forces. Problem-posing is a logical prior task, which allows all previous conceptualizations of a problem to be

treated as questionable. Problematization recognizes that "solutions" are often difficult because the wrong problems are being addressed [in the wrong way]. (Heaney, 1997, p. 12)

Problematization arouses learners to existentially confront and critically evaluate their world, to examine the deeper layers of the symbolic objects before them, and to inquire into the social and political essence of their "taken-for-granted" world (Freire, 1985).

Our attention will now be turned to the complexity of the meanings, motives, and context of an intervention, that is the critical incident, of a worker with her client, which was investigated by Sachs (1987). The analysis will intentionally focus on how the phenomenological investigation of the intervention with the worker opened an essential contradiction in her work. In addition, we will take the opportunity to introduce concepts from other selected parts of our theory base that we believe will be useful to our analysis.

ANALYSIS OF A "TYPICAL" INTERVENTION OF AN INDUSTRIAL SOCIAL WORKER WORKING FOR A LABOR UNION

Introduction

From 1983 to 1987, Sachs (1987) undertook a phenomenological research project aimed at discovering and conceptualizing the precipitates of social work practice interventions. Precipitates include social, interpersonal, and intrapersonal forces that interact at the psychosocial interface. These forces are the meaning and motivational contexts out of which interventions are precipitated. The concept of precipitate is used because it implies a dynamic interactional process between two or more elements that produce change.

The Worker

Sally was a thirty-five-year-old, single, Irish Catholic woman who trained and practiced as a nurse before going on to social work school. She had been working in this, her first job since she received her MSW, for two years. Sally was an alcoholism counselor in the health center of a major international union and was enrolled in an analytic training program.

The Client

Jim was a forty-three-year-old divorced, now remarried, black man with five children. He was referred to the alcoholism clinic after he was found drinking on the job. He had been fired, went to arbitration, and was reinstated under the condition that he get treatment for his drinking.

The Critical Incident

Below is Sally's written description of the critical incident and the initial descriptions of her motives for making the intervention:

> Male, forty-three, black. Recently reinstated at job due to engagement in treatment program. Attendance sporadic but no intervention due to client's health, etc. Arbitration ruled that client must bring in verification of attendance to job weekly. Client informed that counselor will not continue to write verification letter unless client establishes a regular pattern of attendance—given a month in which to do so.

> This intervention was based on the right of a client to choose and accept responsibility for his treatment. Also to accept limits. If client is unable to establish a pattern of attendance, one will be imposed.

The Contradiction and Its Precipitates

Reflecting on Sally's written report and the follow-up interview which was recorded and transcribed, it became clear that two major and contradictory sets of motives were at work precipitating this intervention. Both sets of motives were explicitly or implicitly present in other interventions that Sally reported.

One motivational set centered around Sally's value of client choice and self-determination. Sally wanted clients to be involved in and to own decisions related to their lives and treatment. This was a strongly held personal and professional value. As with all values, this value was overdetermined (Freud, 1900). Like a dream image or symptom (and we add any worker intervention) it has more than one meaning and may express "drives and conflicts from more than one level or aspect [conscious and unconscious, psycho-dynamically and/or socially constructed] of the personality" (Rycroft, 1973, p. 10). For example, Sally believed in the "right of a client to choose to establish a regular pattern of attendance." In her practice experience, she observed that clients did better in treatment when they chose to come. "Somebody who is self motivated [chooses treatment] does much better in the long run. They own it." She also noted that she "didn't want to use coercion" with clients. She believed that "[her] way is not always the right way."

Sally also reported how her life experience influenced her value of choice. "I never owned anything anybody else ever told me. I only believed it if I felt it and wrestled with it. I needed to think about before I owned it, before I took it in and it was mine."

By contrast and in conflict with the value of choice were a set of motivating forces that precipitated Sally's willingness to impose, control, and coerce Jim and other clients. Most important among these forces, in this intervention, appears to be the arbitration judge, who ruled "that client *must* [emphasis ours] bring verification of attendance to job weekly." Observed here is the potent ability of an outside third party, a monitoring institution, to directly control the way in which treatment will proceed. The arbitration judge defined Sally's role as an agent of social control. Critical theory is useful here. It directs attention to "the social structure that shapes and constrains perception as well as the economic forces which determine it" (Findlay, 1978). Once understood, it also directs us to the possibility of changing those structures.

Psychoanalytic theory is also helpful. It would move us to reflect on Sally's report that she "didn't want to use coercion." If there are no negatives in the unconscious (Freud, 1900, 1925/1963d), then we must wonder whether Sally, in her identification with people who used coercion with her, was willing to side, however ambivalently, with an authority who asked her to use coercion with one of the people with whom she worked. Evidence for this is her willingness to "impose" on

Jim. She denied him a verification letter. Here symbolic interaction theory helps us understand how Sally learned to internalize her role as a social control agent and play out the requirements of that role (Mead, 1934; Ohlin, Piven, and Pappenfort, 1956). This placed her in conflict with her professional and personal values.

The motives and meanings of control were not, however, limited to the arbitration judge's ruling. Sally also described being frustrated and angry at Jim. Jim was not a "motivated client." This prevented her from identifying with him and liking him. As a result, Jim had less therapeutic worth (Sachs, 1989) for Sally. The therapeutic worth of a client is predictive of the kind and quality of treatment a worker will provide. Control was, at times, a way for Sally to express her frustration and anger at Jim, a sign of his relative worthlessness as a client.

Sally, however, did not recognize her ambivalence and the contradiction she was in. She denied it and initially blamed Jim for putting her in the controlling role:

> It was [Jim] who put me in that position. He was the one who lost his job and that's why he had to go to the arbitration. If he hadn't lost his job . . . I wouldn't be in this position. Right? . . . I think it's the patient's fault (laughs). He was the winner with the bottle of booze by the side of the cab of the truck.

Though used in the service of rationalization, the above report on how this worker comes to blame a client highlights Ohlin, Piven, and Pappenfort's (1956) observation that a worker, caught between treatment and control functions, is often confused, conflicted, and ambivalent about what is going on and what to do. As a rationalization, however, Sally's report is unconvincing. It did not "fit and work with the data" (Glaser and Strauss, 1967) that Sally had presented. As a result, a phenomenologist aware of the political and economic forces that are at play, that is, a political phenomenologist, must continue to problematize Sally's report and raise questions that will engage Sally in reflection. One way this was done was to ask Sally to reflect on her treatment before and after the request for a verification letter.

Before the request, Sally reported that she allowed Jim to attend sporadically "due to client's health" (Jim had broken his leg). She was willing to do this because "the physical findings on this guy was, was nothing . . . his drinking was problematic but not alcoholic." She believed that Jim "knew the score . . . that if he drank he'd blow it. . . . He knew what he had to do, which was not to drink." Sally believed that Jim "wasn't going to meetings because of physical illness so, you know, at that point, I was ready to let him slide with sporadic phone conversations."

Ironically, it was only when Jim phoned Sally to ask for a verifying letter that she was confronted with the control function that conflicted with her usual treatment orientation and her values. She did not see the control function as being present from the beginning. "In the 'restricted' agency, freedom to pursue the treatment orientation and to reject the control function as a significant part of the worker's role is impossible to achieve" (Ohlin, Piven, and Pappenfort, 1956). The worker will invariably be forced into a contradiction of which he or she may or may not be consciously aware.

After much reflection, Sally arrived at a similar conclusion: "You know, I'll tell you something, . . . because in a lot of job jeopardy cases, of which I have many, to a certain extent it's imposed. I mean, I don't get as hard assed with my voluntary clients."

However, this statement still did not explain why Sally initially denied the influence of the arbitration judge's ruling. That was revealed in Sally's later reflections:

> That's right and I am trying to make them voluntary [clients]. I don't like this discussion. That's what it is, and what frustrates me is they don't start coming here because they want to come, and that's what I want. I want them to come because they want to come. And I hate it when I have to chase them around to tell them they have to come, that they don't have a choice. I don't like it. I do it but I don't like it.

> What immediately comes to mind is that I don't like being told what to do and I don't like telling my clients what they have to do, so, maybe it's easier for me to make it, well, it's his fault because he's caught with the bottle and he has to accept responsibility too. If they're going to tell me what to do, I'm going to tell him what to do. Maybe I xx [xx = tape inaudible] what immediately pops into my head, although I never thought of it before xx. I know, I sense a certain, that I get angry. I mean, I

know that, but I never really thought it through in terms of, well, why do I get angry and what am I angry at and who am I angry at. You know, and very often I assume it's the client that I'm angry at. It's an interesting thing. *I don't like this kind of system* . . . [our emphasis]. Very difficult to, even at times establish relationships because the kinds of limits and requirements.

Through her reflection, Sally was able to consciously observe the contradiction she was caught in for the first time. She was able to analyze and theorize about the contradiction as well as to become clear about its source. She was able to see how the "system" was in conflict with her values and the way she prefers to work. Before this, Sally felt things were "muddy . . . disturbing [and she felt she] didn't know what the hell was going on." She "experimented with various methods and techniques, including client coercion in an attempt to solve [her] work problems" (Ohlin, Piven, and Pappenfort, 1956) and the unconscious contradiction in which she was caught.

How did Sally deal with the contradiction before her rigorous phenomenological reflection made her conscious of it? What might Sally have done with Jim had she been conscious of the contradiction and working from our value, theory, and practice model?

Sally attempted to "solve" the contradiction by trying to get Jim to change his behavior, "accept responsibility for his treatment and accept limits." In effect, Sally's dilemma would be "solved" if Jim behaved differently and chose to control himself. If Jim didn't control himself, then Sally felt justified using control and was willing to impose a pattern of attendance. In this compromise, Sally "satisfies" both the value she places on choice and the arbitration judge's ruling.

Yet Sally also cared about Jim and wanted him to be able to keep his job. She believed a way to do this was to impose restrictions on him that would force him to come to treatment. Sally also said she prefers to work at least once a week with clients and, even prior to the request for a letter, she reported that she was "getting ready to do something, but [she] didn't know what in terms of making a demand that he do something to show that he's involved." The need for a letter in this light reinforced other control motives that were already operative. The unequaled potency of the arbitration judge's demand for a verification letter on Sally's intervention is made clear in her description of how she would work if the letter was not required:

> It influences my interventions a lot, because if I had this guy, for instance, I would work with him somewhat differently, if I didn't have to write these letters. I'm sure that, to begin with, in the beginning I could get him to see me once a week, I mean once a month, in a pretty noncoercive kind of way xx non-threatening kind of way. I think I could kind of invite him to come in to see me once a month. Just to check in, see how he's doing, without him feeling it to be that I'm coming down on him. . . . What I'm saying is I'd work at my own pace. I'd regear to what I feel the client is ready for.

Additional Comments

This example has important implications for practice. Workers need to recognize that restrictive and coercive social institutional forces play a role in precipitating their practice in almost all agency settings. Even in "highly professional" mental health clinics and hospitals, workers described how new fee schedules or mandatory attendance policies imposed from above became major coercive forces in their practice. For example, an article in *The Wall Street Journal* (Jeffrey, 1998) reported on how managed care requirements compromised and subverted a psychiatrist's values and professional judgment about continuing hospital treatment. His willingness to have his severely depressed patient discharged from the hospital was precipitated by his concern that his group might lose an insurance contract. The early discharge led to the patient's suicide attempt. On reflection, he asked, "Was my clinical decision influenced by my not wanting to spend the money for a few extra hospital days? . . . I think my judgment probably was affected" (Jeffrey, 1998, p. 5).

Another worker in a large mental health clinic reported her concerns with a client after her agency raised and changed their fee policy:

> A classic example is that issue with that other client. You know I really found myself wanting to give her the benefit of

the doubt, really wanting to get this kid back in treatment 'cause the kid needed it, and I realized that I was responding on different levels, that administratively I realized that I was going to be up the creek when this client was back in with fee arrears and that things haven't been resolved after clinically, supposedly I had dealt with it and and worked it out with the client. On another level, kind of feeling a little angry at the client for putting me in this position. . . .

I was really going to have to account for it. . . . I mean anybody looking in on it, . . . whether their . . . perspective was administrative [or clinical] so that the two don't always mesh and yet we act as if they do here. That there's a real feeling that, you know, that what makes good clinical sense, you know, is what administratively makes sense too, and sometimes it doesn't. And it gets me in a bind or whatever.

Ironically, the agency contended that workers who questioned the new fee policy had problems of countertransfence that needed to be worked out in their own treatment.

Unfortunately, like Sally, workers are differentially aware and are often willing to rationalize the influence of these coercive forces even when they contradict a worker's personal and professional principles and values. Too often, workers blame the client/victim rather than take on a system that oppresses both the worker and the client.

What a phenomenological investigation can do, as it did with Sally, is to help workers become existentially aware of the variety of forces that interact and conflict to precipitate the work they do. In addition, the method, if used with clients, might also help clients understand their position in the world more clearly. The phenomenological method has the potential to be a tool that will bring greater awareness to practice and perhaps, as Sally would have it, greater choice. Minimally, our approach would require Sally to identify, problematize, and dialogue with Jim about his situation and the social control role that she has in relation to him. This could lead to a conscientization—a "process in which people [Sally and Jim] informed by a critical approach reflect together on their shared experiences as they struggle to change conditions" (Findlay, 1978,

p. 60). Sally, in dialogue with Jim, could then play her role, refuse her role, or, most preferred from our standpoint, work with Jim to change her role, for example, by engaging, perhaps with Jim, her agency, and the arbitration judge.

The problematization of reality allows for and fosters a new perception of the world that can lead to projects of social change (Freire, 1985):

> The longer the problematization proceeds, and the more the subjects enter into the "essence" of the problematized object, the more they are able to unveil this essence. The more they unveil it, the more their awakening consciousness deepens, thus leading to the "conscientization" of the situation by the poorer classes. Their critical self-insertion into reality, that is, their conscientization, makes the transformation of their state of apathy into . . . a viable project. (Freire, 1985, p. 59)

Psychodynamic theory also sheds light on how Sally arrived at an alcohol treatment unit to work with Jim and other clients. Her father was alcoholic. "I don't know whether, because it's my symbolic way of helping him. . . ." Observed here is how a worker's life history affected her choice of work. It is a small step to recognize the need to explore how Sally's countertransference may have affected her work with Jim and the contradiction she was in. Finally, critical theory would necessitate looking at other issues that were not touched. These include cross-racial issues, issues related to ethnicity, the role of the union, social class issues, professional issues, the equality of worker and client, and economic and social justice issues.

Obviously, drinking and driving remains an issue in this case. It also should be problematized as part of the work with Jim, preferably in the context of a group of his fellow drivers who might come to be in a group with Sally. In this context, Jim and other workers can explore the meanings of drinking, both personally and politically. This work would best be done if Sally's role remains that of a social worker and not a social control agent.

Chapter 4

Freud

Psychodynamic and psychoanalytic theories provide a powerful set of concepts for analyzing unconscious ideas, structures, and processes that can facilitate a deeper understanding (conscientization) of individuals in their world. We present several psychodynamic and psychoanalytic ideas and concepts that are useful to deepen the understanding of case material and particularly of workers and clients who meet together as Subjects. We make no attempt to cover all of psychodynamic and psychoanalytic theory (this would be fruitless and silly in such a short volume). We do cover some selected ideas and concepts that are grounded in our practice, reports of case material, student process recordings, and in-class discussions and role plays that will be useful for our project. We recognize that this is not the first time psychodynamic and psychoanalytic ideas have been used by social theorists and clinicians to bring a deeper understanding to the interaction between individuals and groups, and social, economic, and political forces (see, for example, Marcuse, 1966, 1966; Fromm, 1965; Fanon, 1967). We will draw on these and other theorists and clinicians as needed to illuminate these interactions.

We also note the conservative nature of some psychodynamic and psychoanalytic concepts and ideas, particularly some of Freud's stereotyped and culture-bound ideas about the psychology of women and Jung's racist ideas about Jews and people of color. Though we will not deal with them, we note that they fail the test of scientific inquiry and contradict our values of economic and political justice for all people. We, therefore, exclude them from our theory.

LISTENING AND THE UNCONSCIOUS

The most important prayer emerging from the Torah, the Jewish bible, repeated each day, often several times a day, begins with the

Hebrew word "Shema," which means "listen." One of Zen Buddhism's most famous koans, questions for students to meditate on, asks, "What is the sound of one hand clapping?" A student of Zen may spend many years carefully learning to listen fully for the answer. Listening carefully is essential for psychodynamic and psychoanalytic work, for dialogue, and a major practice principle in bridging the false dichotomy between clinical work and social action.

In psychodynamic and psychoanalytic work, one listens to the manifest meanings presented in consciously expressed words and to the silences between words that express themselves as introspection and/or resistance. But workers must also listen for the latent meanings, that is, unconscious meanings, that words and silences express. These can be expressed either in metaphor, in double entendres, in forgetting, in slips of the tongue, and in other ways that reveal ideas and experiences that have been defended against and repressed. They are removed from consciousness because the conflict, anxiety, and pain connected to them would be too much for a person to bear consciously.

Two major foci of clinical work since Freud have been to make the unconscious conscious and then to work through material that has been kept from consciousness because of trauma, conflict, and anxiety. By doing so, individuals develop a deeper and clearer understanding of their motives and themselves as they engage others and their social world. People will then be able to make more fully informed choices about their behavior in the world. These informed choices are essential for authentic self-determination to take place. For Freud and many early analysts, this meant uncovering repressed early experiences from childhood, primarily with parents or primary caretakers. In this way, both the worker and client gain an understanding of how repressed traumas, conflicts, and anxieties of this early period continue to express themselves unconsciously in ways that affect the world of the adult. Infrequently alluded to, and even less frequently engaged by workers or analysts, are the effects of the child's social, economic, and political world. The social, economic, and political world also generate and are filled with traumas, conflicts, and anxieties that have been repressed in childhood. Psychological defenses are similarly marshaled to keep them under repression. Full listening for unconscious material reveals not only repressed ideas and experiences related to one's family and caretakers but also repressed ideas and experiences that emerge from the sociopolitical and economic world of people. In both cases, we believe, "attention must be paid."

It is our experience that making these ideas, experiences, and dynamics conscious will frequently expose contradictions. The avoidance of this material is itself a contradiction to the work of psychodynamic and psychoanalytic therapy that is aimed at uncovering *all* unconscious material.

Franz Fanon (1967) was an important writer, psychoanalyst, and theorist who amplified this theme. In *Black Skins, White Masks* he presents a dream of a "Negro":

> I had been walking for a long time, I was extremely exhausted, I had the impression that something was waiting for me, I climbed barricades and walls, I came to an empty hall, and from behind the door I heard noise. In this second room there were white men, and I found that I too was white. (p. 99)

In analyzing this dream, Fanon, the traditional clinician, argues that the dreamer must be made conscious of his inferiority complex and his desire for whitening. "As a [political] psychoanalyst," he realizes that he must also:

> help my patient . . . to act in the direction of a change in the social structure. . . . Because he lives in a society that makes his inferiority complex possible, in a society that derives its stability from the perpetuation of this complex, in a society that proclaims the superiority of one race; to the identical degree to which that society creates difficulties for him, he will find himself thrust into a neurotic situation. (p. 100)

Fanon observes that dreams depend not only on our instincts, Eros and Thanatos, and early object relations, but also on the contents of the culture and society in which dreamers find themselves. These include, most importantly, the cultural and societal norms, values, and beliefs about race, class, and gender. It is these contents that determine how the instincts will express themselves (Fanon, 1967).

A study by Lieberman (1988) adds weight to Fanon's ideas. She explored the proposition that people develop unconscious internal representations of community. Using dream content related to community, she uncovered associations suggesting that people internalize the social institutional world, including the political economy. The social institutional world is a powerful unconscious addition to the overdetermined symbols that make up dreams.

Some analysts might contend that all of the social symbols and meanings have, at their root, a sexual or aggressive meaning. These meanings are not denied. As with conflict-free and conflict-filled spheres of the ego (Hartman, 1958), however, there are conflict-filled and conflict-free spheres of the social institutional world. These exist from infancy and have been internalized through a child's interactions with his or her parents and significant others who represent the social institutional world. To gain a full understanding and make a full interpretation, a worker must acknowledge not only the instinctual and early object world of the individual, but also the social institutional world. That world interacts in significant, sometimes traumatic, ways with the instinctual world and determines the contents of the instinctual and object world.

In the unconscious, the instinctual forces (libidinal and aggressive), the processes (e.g., displacement, projection), and the objects (e.g., therapist or friend) related to such things as race, class, and gender may be mobile and transferable. However, the contents of the unconscious, that is, how one experiences, values, feels one ought to act toward, and believes about, are filled with specific content related to race, class, and gender.

Contemporaneously involved with the early gratification and/or frustration of the instincts in relation to early parental and caretaking objects, these contents of the social, economic, and political world of the individual have been internalized and remain, in part, unconscious. Erich Fromm elaborates on this idea in his discussion of the "social unconscious":

> Freud'[s unconscious] was mainly concerned with individual repression, the student of Marxist social psychology will be most concerned with the "social unconscious." This concept refers to that repression of inner reality which is common to large groups. Every society must make every effort not to permit its members (or those of a particular class) to be aware

of impulses which, if they were conscious, could lead to socially "dangerous" thoughts or actions. Effective censorship occurs, not at the level of the printed or spoken word, but by preventing thoughts from even becoming conscious, that is, by preventing dangerous awareness. . . . The repressed impulse must be kept under repression and replaced by ideologies which deny it or affirm its opposite. The bored, anxious, unhappy man of today's industrial society is taught to think that he is happy and full of fun. . . . In some systems love of life is repressed and love of property is cultivated instead. . . . (1966, pp. 239-240)

LISTENING TO THE UNCONSCIOUS OF WORKERS AND STUDENTS

Good listening also applies to supervisors as they listen to workers and students and/or assess student process. For example, a student presented the following process recording:

Hi, Meg. Before we start chit-chatting today, I want to let you know that our financial wizard Linda is free after our session today. And I know that you and I had talked briefly about this before, and I think it's helpful for you to talk to her so the two of you can figure out the best way to make paying for sessions more manageable.

Here the student's "chit-chatting" seems to diminish the importance of her therapeutic talk with Meg and raises the importance of the discussion of payment for sessions. Clearly, her supervisor, representing the agency, had penetrated the worker's unconscious and made important what was important to the agency, namely payment.

Another student in the class stimulated by this discussion recognized how her anger about money issues was sometimes displaced onto her work with a client. She reported:

I just want to speak to another way in which financial concerns play into the therapeutic relationship, and that is that we talked a lot about the worker [being] pressured by the agency to talk about money. I know in situations where I've had clients that haven't paid, and the agency's billing department has come to me, and come to me, I've resented the client, because I would have definitely had feelings directed toward the clients that were doing this and that I had to keep bringing up the issue, which was uncomfortable for both of us and that gets acted out in treatment. But that's a part that hasn't really been brought into this.

The displacement of anger, due to the worker's discomfort (anxiety) in the above example, is not unusual and may be on the increase as agencies are threatened by the bottom lines of managed care systems, whose profits are more important than people.

It is beyond the scope of this chapter to discuss in depth why ideas about the unconscious and its relationship to the social structure have been neglected. However, part of the answer may lay in Fanon's (1967) suggestion that analysts would, by recognizing the impact of the social institutional structure, have to engage in efforts to change that structure and their own privileged position in that structure. As Freire (1989a) points out:

> Well-intentioned professionals . . . eventually discover that certain of their educational failures must be ascribed, not to the intrinsic inferiority of the "simple men [sic] of the people," but to the violence of their own act[s]. . . . Divesting themselves of and renouncing their myths represents, at that moment, an act of self violence. (pp. 154-155)

In psychodynamic terms, to avoid this experience of self-violence and the anxiety that attends it, professionals mobilize defenses such as denial, rationalization, or projection. This, as Marx (1844/1978) suggests, comes with the price of the "alienation of [the worker's] labor":

> . . . it does not belong to his [sic] essential being; that in his work, therefore, he does not affirm himself but denies himself, does not feel content but unhappy, does not develop freely his physical and mental energy but mortifies his body and ruins his mind. The worker therefore only feels himself outside his

work, and in his work he feels outside himself. . . . His labor is therefore not voluntary, but coerced; it is forced labor. It is therefore not the satisfaction of a need; it is merely a means to satisfy needs external to it. (pp. 110-111)

The increasingly coercive and alienating affects of managed care on workers are well described in Marx's observations.

THE REAL AND THE RESISTANCE

In the previous example related to fees, students rightly pointed out that some clients may be using nonpayment as a "real" resistance to treatment rather than "really" being unable to pay. Both of course can be true simultaneously and each would need to be dealt with in its own right. That a fee was too high would then be the hook in reality that would need to be acknowledged to the client so that whatever unconscious issues were being played out could then be dealt with. As Gill (1980) pointed out, the hook in reality, real or plausible, often needs to be addressed before addressing the unconscious meaning. Each meaning, real or imagined, whether conscious or unconscious, it should be added, can and often does illuminate the other.

In the above case, the meanings of money, to the worker and the client, would be important subjects. Money would have meanings for each of them related to their early experiences in their families, but also meanings related to the political economy as they experienced it with their families, and currently in the world in which they live. We would also want to note parenthetically that medical care and money have different meanings, consciously and unconsciously, for poor families, middle-class families, and rich families, depending on whether they have health insurance. Money would also have a different meaning for similar families who lived in a country with a universal national health program. Finally, money would have yet different meanings to workers in these situations who engage these families and to managed care administrators.

The mission statement of the agency in which this example took place included a statement of willingness to "treat people regardless of their ability to pay." This example reveals a contradiction between the agency's mission and its treatment of both workers and clients. To the extent that this mission is not followed with other clients, there is an opportunity to bring other workers and their clients together for social action in the agency.

When the above contradiction was pointed out in a role play, the student who played the client expressed the following:

> And I was really trying to get into the role, and I was feeling down on myself, and oppressed, and really down on myself. And when you presented that contradiction to me for the first time, I got angry. And I felt angry at the agency. I put it outside myself. So that was really good for me in that role. . . . And at that point it really got refocused for me as anger at the agency. So that was good.

Hence, anger, initially internalized against the self, can be, through conscientization, directed to its proper place, that is, to the agency that is in contradiction with itself. Making the contradiction within the agency conscious might allow anger to be appropriately directed outward. This would free the worker's and client's energy, consumed in anger directed inward, for greater productive introspection. Dealing with the real money issue should not prevent a worker from dealing with unconscious issues related to money or resistance about paying fees. The source of this resistance may be, and often is, related to anxiety about expressing anger at a worker or an agency about other issues, such as a worker's slighting the client, or a secretary mistreating the client. Dealing with fees on a social action level would be a parameter (Eissler, 1953) in the treatment that would need to be acknowledged.

NEGATION

In his 1925 paper "Negation," Freud tells us that

> the subject matter of a repressed image or thought can make its way into consciousness on the condition that it is denied. Negation is a way of taking account of what is repressed; indeed, it is actually a removal of the repression, though not, of course, an acceptance of what is repressed. . . .

A negative judgment is the intellectual substitute for repression; the "No" in which it is expressed is the hall-mark of repression, a certificate of origin. . . . By the help of negation, the thinking process frees itself from the limitations of repression, and enriches itself with subject-matter without which it could not work efficiently. (1925/1963d, pp. 213-214)

A student reported an African-American client in a mental hospital telling him that "it doesn't matter anyway what I say, nobody cares." He was speaking of how workers talk to black folks. We opened this negation in the context of our class discussion of language in relation to race and how language has penetrated the culture and is used by people, including workers and students, in ways that might be unconsciously offensive. This led to a student presenting a case related to the issue of race.

The case, shared by a young white man, was that of a twenty-seven-year-old African-American woman named Alberta:

She came in a wheelchair. One of the first things she said to me is that she had been a medical student. Everyone on staff were determined to negate that, to say it wasn't true. And my thought was [that it was] because she was black. That was one thing, and the other thing was that she would never look people in the eye, that was a very big issue with the treatment team, basically they didn't keep in mind anything that was cultural, is my sense. Her diagnosis, one of them was borderline, so they called her *big B* and that was an easy way to label her, and label patients. . . . So when I met with her it was a similar experience—she didn't look me in the eye, she didn't talk to me, things like that. I brought it up to my supervisor, the cultural piece, she didn't go with it, wasn't interested. And then I, it was my first month there, and I was gun-shy, scared to speak up. This is where the contradiction was. I knew something wrong was going on, and this was not the only patient this was happening to, by any means, and we'd have treatment team sessions and all these things would be brought out and discussed and discussed and I never said anything. It turns out that we had a family meeting with her and the case manager and my supervisor regarding her discharge and it came out that many things typical of borderline personalities came out. She could never decide on anything, the onus would be on her to make decisions, things like that. The contradiction for me was that the treatment team was in some ways correct in how they looked at the patient, in other ways they were far off. So there was inordinate racism in my opinion, I constantly struggled whether to bring that up, and never did.

One of the authors attempted to focus the student more concretely on his interaction with Alberta. He asked whether Alberta said anything else other than that she was a medical student. The student answered that, "She would tell me that her friends at home would get upset at her when she would become suicidal." He added that "She knew medical terms and the staff couldn't explain that," but were dismissive and that staff said, "She [was] lying about some things."

At this point, one of the authors pointed out that there were at least two levels of relationship. The first was the student's relationship with staff and the second his relation with Alberta. "Lots of information about the staff but little about your interaction with Alberta." The author again asked if there was "any information that Alberta gave, in relation to him, that would indicate that, explicitly or implicitly, she was picking something up herself [about racism]":

> Yeah, in one of first meetings with her. She said that other worker asked whether she was on welfare or been raised by single mother. She said that they always do this to black folk or something like that. And again I talked to my supervisor about it and she [the supervisor] dismissed that.

The teacher then inquired further, "You spoke to your supervisor about it, but did you speak to Alberta about it when she raised it, or was that another example of your avoiding it?" The student answered that "I did say, sort of empathized and said, 'sounds really hard' and then I think she said, dismissing her own feeling, 'It doesn't matter anyway what I say. Nobody cares.'"

Examining Alberta's negation of her voice and her feeling that no one cares, it would be important for the worker to understand just how important it is for her to be heard and for someone to care. Her need to deny its importance also needs to be understood as partly connected to the pain she endures when not being listened to, and the staff's dismissal of what she says. The staff describe her not as fully human, but a "big B," i.e., borderline personality. It is ironic, but not surprising, that the medical staff confirmed her pathology by suggesting that Alberta did not look them straight in the eye. Rather than seeing her as a whole person with a culture of her own, they dehumanized her.

In practice, the student might, at the very least, send a message that he cares, that it is important to care, and that Alberta's wish appears to be that someone does care. He might then venture an interpretation that she, in fact, seems to care and that if she did care, her experience of the staff's not caring would be painful. This would explain and make it understandable why she says she "doesn't care." The worker could ask a question about "what it might mean" for Alberta "to care." If she could accept her wish for caring, the worker might then move to what they might want to do together about the lack of caring at the hospital.

If Alberta could not engage at this point, the worker could raise the issue of caring at the next case conference or staff meeting. The workers at the agency would then be forced to deal with the issue of what it means to care and Alberta's need for them to do so. It is worth noting that the student listened to his client but did nothing to expose this issue to the staff. He gave us evidence that his own anxiety (see his reference to being "gun-shy") was too great at the time. Here, a Freirian supervisor might productively be supportive and talk to the student's unconscious castration anxiety by assuring him that he would be supported and not cut off if and when he chose to bear witness.

Ideally, the student could use Alberta's negation about not caring as a way of talking with the other staff about caring for Alberta and other clients. He could point to the contradiction that exists in their work. Specifically, these workers voiced values related to listening and cultural sensitivity yet acted in ways that were dismissive and not culturally sensitive. A staff may choose to use rationalization, a frequent maneuver among professional staff, to deny that their behavior is anything but culturally sensitive and blame the victim/patient for being so paranoid and crazy. They may also blame the student for being "too sensitive," thus negating the fact that sensitivity is an important professional value.

Negation by staff may have also been a way to deal with the contradictions that existed related to issues of race and culture within the agency. The agency was vulnerable; it had almost no minority staff. It would be painful for staff to open this contradiction and easier to keep it under repression, along with whatever unconscious individual racism existed in agency workers and administrators. Repression would also keep the institutional racism that exists in the agency's structure under wraps. This institutional racism would be in contradiction to the to the agency's mission and the workers' values. It is too often the case that students and workers who raise these issues, that is, are the messengers, are "shot." Our student may have had good reason to be "gun-shy." It is important to be able to distinguish between rational and irrational paranoia.

Negation in the Class

Negation is also evident among professors. One of the authors suggested to the class that "there was certainly no demand that this [model] becomes the way that everyone has to do it." Clearly his wish was that it would be. To be fully honest he would need to acknowledge his wish and plead, as he wrote in the Bertha Capen Reynolds newsletter, "guilty your honor, but not guilty enough" (Newdom, 1997).

CLINICAL NEUTRALITY

There is a notion that clinical work is, or should be, neutral, and that this neutrality needs to be maintained. Many clinicians see social action as not neutral. Doing social action, in this view, contaminates the clinical process, makes transference impossible, is a sign of countertransference in the worker, and prevents the unconscious from unfolding. To illustrate, a student in a role play, playing a supervisor, said:

> Well . . . I think, my concern is that you're getting into it [social activism] to the exclusion of what our education is really about,

which is clinical work. And I think that it is important to look from a personal perspective at what your need is to focus on the advocacy, to focus almost exclusively on the advocacy for the client. . . . My work with you is to address the clinical issues. And while I want to sort of support you a little bit on the advocacy stuff, but I really, I think we need to explore why you're leaning toward that . . .

Another student playing the supervisor added that she was aware that the student is an eldest child, and that advocacy with a client was similar to taking on the needs and assuming responsibility for others in the student's family of origin. We suggest that these interventions by the "supervisors" are also not neutral but political and favor a particular type of political work with the client, that is, work that maintains the status quo.

Our position is that neutrality is not possible in social work or in any of the human services and that progressive politics, rooted in a clear value system, are preferred. "It's naive to consider [the role of social worker] as abstract in a matrix of neutral methods and techniques for action that doesn't take place in neutral reality" (Freire, 1985, p. 39). Workers have many intervention options for what a client brings to treatment. There are choices to be made about whether to focus on a client's individual troubles, real or imagined by the worker, or to open the full spectrum of a client's experiences, including his or her relation to the social institutional structure.

There are reactionary and progressive social workers. Reactionary social workers "assist in the 'normalization' of the 'established order' which serves the power elite's interests" (Freire, 1985, p. 39). For example, a worker who describes a client's anger only in pathological terms and does not recognize the hook in social reality of the client that may belie a partial healthy expression of emotions is negating some of the client's experience. Progressive social workers, on the other hand:

> are interested in individuals developing a critical view of reality. . . . Through their own thought and actions, people can see the conditioning of perception in their social structure, and in this way their perception begins to change. . . . It is important to see that social reality can be transformed; that it is made by

men [*sic*] and can be changed by men; that it is not something untouchable. . . . (Freire, 1985, p. 39)

In this view, all of what a client brings to the therapeutic process can be looked at critically, both individual troubles and social issues. "This change of perception, which occurs in the 'problematizing' of a reality in conflict, in viewing our problems in life in their true context, requires us to reconfront our reality" (Freire, 1985, p. 40).

ANXIETY

We end this chapter with a brief review of some of Freud's (1926/1959, 1932/1965) ideas about the affective state of anxiety. In relation to the origin and meaning of anxiety, Freud was characteristically deeply reflective and changed his views over a period of more than thirty-five years:

> The deeper we penetrate into the study of mental processes the more we recognize their abundance and complexity. A number of simple formulas which to begin with seemed to meet our needs have later turned out to be inadequate. . . . Here, where we are dealing with anxiety everything is in a state of flux and change. . . . I cannot promise that it will have been settled to our satisfaction, but it is to be hoped that we shall have made a little progress. (1932/1965, pp. 92-93)

In his last major writing on anxiety, Freud (1932/1965), having developed his structural theory, put forward the idea that "the ego is the sole seat of anxiety—that the ego alone can produce and feel anxiety (p. 85). . . ." The precipitates of anxiety are varied.

Most clearly, anxiety can be a reaction to a real situation of external danger. In this situation the ego can prepare to deal with the danger or flee from it. More complicated is anxiety arising from inside the person, anxiety signals that arise from past traumas that were real and repressed, or that emerge in relation to libidinous and aggressive instincts during a child's normal developmental stages. The major templates for traumas related to internal anxiety are: birth, separation anxiety in infancy, male castration anxiety in the phallic stage, a woman's loss of object love in the phallic stage, and loss of love of the superego, that is, moral anxiety, which develops first in latency but can continue developing through an individual's adulthood (Kearney, 1970).

It is impossible to flee from internal anxiety, and individuals deal with this type of anxiety through psychological defenses and symptom formation. This is important for our work since workers who experience anxiety that prevents them from following through on their values often end up in a contradiction. We can see this when workers displace their anger at their agency onto a client. Contradictions grounded in anxiety also occur when workers become depressed because they hold back what they wish to say to a supervisor or in staff meetings. This becomes a signal of anxiety related to rejection or losing love.

Chapter 5

From Positivist Sociology and Social Psychology to Symbolic Interaction Theory

This chapter will complement the chapter on psychoanalytic and psychodynamic theory. We will also highlight connections with phenomenology theory. Specifically, we have discussed how psychoanalytic and psychodynamic theory focus attention on the structures and processes of an individual's unconscious, what Freud termed "the instincts and their vicissitudes" (1915/1963c). Some analysts, such as Fromm (1966), who was also an early critical theorist, as well as Groddeck (1977) and Reich (1946), were well aware of the role of society in shaping personality and behavior. They recognized the power society holds in relation to the individual even at an unconscious level. Freud, in several of his writings and particularly in *Civilization and Its Discontents* (1930/1962a), noted the restraining nature of society and culture on the individual. But his main focus was on the individual's unconscious, the vicissitudes of the instincts, and particularly the role of aggression and guilt in relation to the development of civilization. In spite of his intrapsychic focus, and though he thought that socialism, as a means to do away with the effects of the aggressive instincts, was an "untenable illusion," Freud also wrote in *Civilization and Its Discontents* that:

> Anyone who has tasted the misery of poverty in his own youth and has experienced the indifference and arrogance of the well-to-do, should be safe from the suspicion of having no understanding or good will toward endeavors to fight against the inequality of wealth among men [*sic*] and all that leads to. (1930/1962a, p. 60)

And, later in this monograph, comparing the role of religion or ethics to socialism's ability to temper the aggressive instinct, Freud wrote, "I too think it quite certain that a real change in the relations of human beings to possessions would be of more help than any ethical commands . . ." (p. 90).

Nevertheless, Freud's thesis about society, while tempering an "oversocialized conception of man [sic]," which dominates some sociological theory (Wrong, 1961), represents an overinstinctual-ized conception of human beings. This conception needs tempering by theories that take account of the influence of society, culture, and consciousness in shaping personality and behavior. What we call the contents of a society or culture—social institutions, social roles, and the norms, values, and beliefs that are embedded in and sustain those institutions and roles—predate the individual and a particular individual's biological (including instincts) endowments. These contents interact and affect individuals in unique ways. Through the process of socialization, they play a role, along with biology, in reproducing individuals who will promote and sustain a particular society or culture. This includes a society's contradictions that can lead to social change. We now turn to a selected group of sociological theories, ideas, and concepts. Our objectives are to present accounts related to:

- the development of European sociology beginning with August Comte;
- the beginnings of selected movements in American sociology and particularly the development of the Chicago School of sociology; and
- explore the work of the Chicago School of philosophy, social psychology, and sociology, and particularly the contribution of George Herbert Mead.

AUGUST COMTE'S POSITIVISM AND THE ORIGINS OF EUROPEAN AND AMERICAN SOCIOLOGY

August Comte is credited with being the father of the "science" of sociology. Writing in the aftermath and turmoil of the French Revolution, he saw sociologists as philosopher-priests who would use sociological science to study, understand, bring order to, and control the way society was to move and progress. In the wake of the growing achievements in the natural sciences, the technological advances of the industrial revolution, and the bureaucratization of social, and particularly economic, organizations, he saw the possibility for unlimited progress and a stable social order.

Comte's development of positivism, his utopianism, and his elitism assumed societal progress that Albert Salomon (1955), in a too-neglected work, *The Tyranny of Progress*, suggested helped to pave the way for the development of fascism. Salomon observed similar utopian trends in Marx's sociology that, he suggests, opened the way for Bolshevism and Stalinism. However, Salomon's description of "Comte's religion of humanity [leaves] nothing to the imagination":

> It was a thoroughly grim affair, covering the control of all phases of life, omitting no area of intellectual activity from its dogma down to the smallest details of budget or the press. He even went so far as to draw up a new calendar with positivist saints designated for every day of the year. His early conviction of the negative character of freedom was borne out of the way he elaborated his rules for running a positivist society. (p. 79)

This is a far cry from Marx's view of people and his goals for individual freedom and emancipation:

> In a communist society, where no one has one exclusive sphere of activity, but each can become accomplished in any branch [of life] he wishes, society regulates the general production and thus makes it possible for me to do one thing today and another tomorrow, to hunt in the morning, fish in the afternoon, rear cattle in the evening, criticize [*sic*] after dinner, just as I have a mind, without ever becoming a hunter, fisherman, shepherd or critic. (Marx and Engels, 1970, p. 53)

Unfortunately, utopian theories and theoretical fads promising extraordinary results have penetrated and continue to penetrate social welfare and clinical theory and practice. A brief look at practice journals will display "flavor of the month" brands of quick-fix theories and therapies such as behaviorism, drug therapy, encounter groups, primal scream, constructivism, postmodernism, and so on. Although some of these theories include useful ideas, they often promise more than they can deliver. This is largely because of their unwillingness to acknowledge the complexity of the world and the imperfection of human beings. Workers and students often want to know "the answer" and "the way to fix things" for a client, if not for themselves. Few are willing to "make the [very long] road by walking" (Horton and Freire, 1990), to take the time for deep reflection that too often comes up with less-than-utopian solutions. Clinical work and societal work are interminable (Freud, 1937/1963a).

THE BEGINNINGS OF AMERICAN SOCIOLOGY

The beginnings of American sociology and social psychology at the turn of the century followed Comte's utopian ideas of progress and the need for order. The work of the English social Darwinist Herbert Spencer and his American follower, the sociologist William Graham Sumner, also influenced its development. Where Marx and even Comte saw the potential for progress in the proletariat, Spencer and the American social Darwinists saw salvation and social progress coming from the industrial owning classes. As Hofstadter (1955) wrote:

> Spencer . . . was ultra-conservative. His categorical repudiation of state interference with the "natural," unimpeded growth of society led him to oppose all state aid to the poor. They were unfit, he said, and should be eliminated. "The whole effort of nature is to get rid of such, to clear the world of them, and make room for the better." Nature is as insistent upon fitness of mental character as she is upon physical character. . . . Under nature's laws all alike are put on trial. "If they are sufficiently complete to live, they do live, and it is well that they should live. If they are not sufficiently complete to live, they die and it is best that they should die." (p. 41)

Later, quoting William Graham Sumner, one of the fathers of American sociology, he wrote:

Let it be understood that we cannot go outside this alternative: liberty, inequality, survival of the fittest; not-liberty, equality, survival of the unfittest. The former carries society forward and favors all its best members; the latter carries society downwards and favors its worst members. (p. 51)

Though embedded in the theory itself, social Darwinism was used to justify a set of values that accounted for the "natural selection" of the rich, a practice that promoted laissez-faire individualism, a capitalist approach to economics, and the absence of social reform. These secular values and practices were supported by religious theories and ideas embedded in the Protestant ethic (Weber, 1958). The interests of capitalism were and are currently served by both a secular and a religious theory base embedded in values that would "improve" the species and get the rich to heaven. To make things even more pernicious, the growing eugenics movement of the nineteenth and twentieth centuries added a racial bias to these theories that influenced not only the social Darwinists but also social reformers and former socialists such as Margaret Sanger, who could write that "the chief issue of birth control [is] more children from the fit, less from the unfit" (quoted in Davis, 1983, pp. 213-214). Lest anyone believe this thinking has lost its force in American values, theory, policy, and practice, we would refer the reader to the works of Gilder (1981), Murray (1984), and Herrnstein and Murray (1994) and to policies related to the rights of immigrants, welfare recipients, unions, and so on.

There were, however, other theorists and theories. Among these was Lester Ward, who disagreed with Spencer's social Darwinism and natural law and attacked Sumner's formulations about laissez-faire. He emphasized the differences between biology and social behavior, maintained an allegiance to Comte, and promoted the need for positivist science to have a role in government policymaking so that social progress could be ensured. Of the differences between himself and the laissez-faire economists, Ward wrote:

The opposing positive school of economists simply demands an opportunity to utilize the social forces for human advantage in precisely the same manner that the physical forces have been utilized. It is only through artificial control of natural phenomena that science is made to minister to human needs; and if social laws are really analogous to physical laws, there is no reason why social science may not receive practical applications such as have been given to physical science. (quoted in Hofstadter, 1955, p. 73)

Although Ward was a social planner with reformist ideas that promoted equal opportunity and influenced socialists, he was no socialist himself. He did, however, interact with and/or was followed by religious and secular reformers, socialists, the pragmatists, social psychologists, and symbolic interactionists from the Chicago School. It was these developments in sociology and social psychology that set the American stage for the mostly Jewish actors of the Frankfurt School, the critical theorists, and the social phenomenologists, when they arrived in the United States from Nazi Germany. But we are now ahead of ourselves.

Late-nineteenth-century America began to show the strains and contradictions of unbridled capitalism in the form of two major depressions and economic panics (Hofstadter, 1955). These upheavals were fertile soil for the development of labor unions, such as the Knights of Labor and the Industrial Workers of the World, and religious reformers who, while not socialists, did want social reform, and an end to the worst abuses of laissez-faire capitalism and the atheistic ideas of social Darwinism.

Yet some utopian ideas remained. For example, in popular books such as Bellamy's *Looking Backward* (1888), there were strong arguments against competition and for "the Brotherhood of Humanity, one of the eternal truths that govern the world's progress on lines that distinguish human nature from brute nature" (quoted in Hofstadter, 1955, p. 113).

Early American socialists sometimes attempted to have it both ways. They rejected Spencer's ideas about individualism while trying to keep his theory as it related to social evolution and, with the understanding of sudden biological mutations, revolutionary change (Hofstadter, 1955). Later, more independent socialists, such as William English Walling, combined socialism with the humanism of pragmatism, noting that:

the control of life around us matters less than the control of our own lives, and the control of our physiological evolution less than our psychological evolution and of social progress. (quoted in Hofstadter, 1955, p. 118)

In pragmatism, there was a new emphasis on experimentation with the uses of knowledge. Ideas embraced by pragmatism were freedom, control of the environment, flexibility in social thought, humanism in values and outlook, an emphasis on empirical exploration, novelty in the universe, induction, probability, and indeterminacy.

In William James, who, with John Dewey, was the chief proponent of pragmatism in America, we find the pluralist who abhorred the absolutism of Spencer. He believed that moral judgments require some minimal uncertainty and that human beings must be active agents in the world.

Theories and knowledge were no longer to be set out as absolute truths but were to be tested. What is present in James' thinking is the development of ideas that would fit well with critical practice:

> Every actually existing consciousness seems to itself at any rate to be a fighter for ends, of which many, but for its presence, would not be ends at all. Its powers of cognition are mainly subservient to these ends, discerning which facts further them and which do not. (quoted in Hofstadter, 1955, p. 132)

Although Hofstadter suggests James was somewhat slow to social reform and bound up with individualism, he also indicates that in his later years James expressed his belief in "some sort of socialistic equilibrium" (1955, p. 135).

Dewey, who taught at the University of Chicago, was influenced by Ward's social reformism and James' critique of Spencer. In a powerful departure from laissez-faire theorists, he believed that "direct participation in events is necessary to genuine understanding" (Hofstadter, 1955, p. 138). This formulation anticipates Freire, who, as an educator, was certainly acquainted with Dewey's work. Dewey was a social reformer whose theory had a base in liberal democratic values and was susceptible to change based on experience. It was a social psychological theory that took account not only of an individual's personality but also an individual's social surroundings. As a social activist, he wrote:

We may desire abolition of war, industrial justice, greater equality of opportunity for all. But no amount of preaching good will or the golden rule or cultivation of sentiments of love and equality will accomplish the results. There must be change in objective arrangements and institutions. We must work on the environment, not merely on the hearts of men. (quoted in Hofstadter, 1955, p. 160)

The theories of social reformers have also had their moments of ascendancy in American social policy and social practice. This was particularly true during the depression of the 1930s and the Great Society programs of the late 1960s. Though their influence has been on the decline for the past three decades, there are echoes and elaboration in the voices of elected officials such as Senator Paul Wellstone, Congresswoman Maxine Waters, Congressman Bernie Sanders, activists including Cheri Honkala and Dennis Rivera and social welfare critics and writers such as Cloward, Piven, Withorn, Dujon, Blau, and Abramovitz, among others.

Dewey was a philosophical pragmatist. He was also, along with his colleagues George Herbert Mead and Charles Horton Cooley, a social psychologist. The sociological theory that grew out of the work of these thinkers came to be known as symbolic interaction theory. It is to the contributions of these theorists and to the sociology practiced at the University of Chicago that we now turn.

SYMBOLIC INTERACTION THEORY AND THE CHICAGO SCHOOL OF SOCIOLOGY

Symbolic interaction theory places society at the center of understanding. It is in society that human beings, who have the capability to reflect on themselves and others, are socialized. In society, people develop minds and a self. Society is also where they learn, first through gestures and later through play and games using symbolic language, to internalize social roles and to enact those roles in social groups and social institutions. Society, for Mead, who labeled himself a social behaviorist, became the counterweight to Freudian theorists. Mead (1934) called Freud's theory a "fantastic psychology"* that saw society emerging from individual biology, that is, the vicissitudes of a person's instinctual life.

Other contrasts are also significant and important complements to Freud's ideas. Mead was concerned with an individual's consciousness and paid little if any attention to the powerful effects of unconscious motivations. Though paying attention to early childhood and the beginnings of the socialization process, Mead also recognized that adult socialization and experience could play a significant role in human development. In this respect, he was more socially but less biologically deterministic than was Freud's instinct-based psychology.

But Mead was never a strict social determinist and, as C. Wright Mills suggests, his concept of the "I," similar to:

> Freud's "Id," Marx's "Freiheit," [and] Karen Horney's "spontaneity" lie . . . against the triumph of the alienated man [*sic*]. They are trying to find some center in man-as-man which would enable them to believe that in the end he cannot be made into, that he cannot finally become, such an alien creature—alien to nature, to society, to self. (Mills, 1961, p. 172)

Again, we will use those parts of theory which are useful to our understanding of society and human phenomena, those which do not contradict our values. For example, we would not include Mead's comparisons of children with so-called "primitive societies" or Cooley's (1964) racist idea that, "It is true, no doubt, that there are differences in race capacity, so great that a large part of mankind are possibly incapable of any kind of social organization. . . ." (p. 159). We use theory that can be synthesized in a complementary way into our value and theory base, for example, concepts that triumph over alienation (Mills, 1961).

Rather than debating the weight that each theory or concept should carry, we prefer to use those theoretical ideas which do not contradict our values or do serious injury to other concepts and ideas we use. For example, we believe that Freud's ideas about unconscious processes enhance our understanding of human mo-

---

*Freud would, no doubt, take pleasure in Mead's put-down, recognizing the unconscious compliment in what Mead was saying.

tivation and behavior and must be blended with Mead's ideas about the role society plays in human development. In this spirit, we will explore some of the central concepts and ideas Mead developed in his classic *Mind, Self, and Society* (1934).

As a Darwinist, but not a social Darwinist, Mead saw the evolutionary process in the ability of human beings to develop minds that could not only engage in a conversation of gestures, as would two dogs who respond to each other's growls, but for these gestures to become shared significant symbols, the most important of which is language:

> Gestures become significant when they implicitly arouse in the individual making them the same responses which they explicitly arouse, or are supposed to arouse, in other individuals, the individuals to whom they are addressed; and in all conversation of gestures, within the social process, whether external (between different individuals) or internal (between a given individual and himself [*sic*]), the individual's consciousness of the content and the flow of meaning involved depends on his thus taking the attitude of the other toward his gestures. . . .

> Only in terms of gestures as significant symbols is the existence of mind or intelligence possible; for only in terms of gestures which are significant symbols can thinking—which is simply an internalized or implicit conversation of the individual with himself by means of gestures—take place. The internalization in our experience of the external conversation of gestures which we carry on with other individuals in the social process is the essence of thinking; and the gestures thus internalized are significant symbols because they have the same meaning for all individual members of a given society or social group. . . . (Mead, 1934, p. 47)

It is shared meanings that allow an individual to take the role of the other and imagine with some accuracy what the other's reactions will be to their significant gestures, behaviors, and actions. In this way, an individual's actions can be intentional. These intentions can be accurately predictive of the future behavior of the other (as they have been created from the individual's past social experiences). Shared social meanings will be reinforced, and a relatively cooperative society is made possible. This is very much like Schutz's taken-for-granted world and why Berger and Luckmann (1966) in *The Social Construction of Reality* were comfortable moving between social phenomenology and symbolic interaction theory.

In addition, individuals are able to "take themselves as objects" and to reflect and make judgments about themselves. For Mead (1934), "mind is the reflective intelligence of the human animal" (p. 118). Reflectivity is essential to understanding the praxis described by Freire.

From the development of mind, Mead moved to the more inclusive development of the self which "arises in the process of social experience and activity, that is, develops in the given individual as a result of his [*sic*] relations to that process as a whole and to other individuals within that process" (p. 136).

The self, for Mead, has two aspects, the "I" and the "me." The "I" is the unique, spontaneous, not quite predictable part of the self that can surprise itself. It brings uncertainty to social situations (Strauss, 1956). "The 'I' is the response of the organism to the attitudes of others. . . . The attitudes of the others constitute the organized 'me'" (Mead, 1934, p. 175). It is the "I" that reacts to the "me" at any moment but the "me," which is always there, that remembers what the "I" has done and, representing the attitudes of others, makes judgments.

The "me" develops in children's play where individuals learn to take the role and attitude of the other, for example, mother, father, teacher, and so on. The "me" then becomes the set of attitudes and expectations of the other. Later, as the child learns games (whether baseball or family life) where there is more than one role, and therefore more than one set of attitudes, the child learns to hold a variety of attitudes simultaneously. This, Mead (1934) called "the generalized other":

> The generalized other represents the attitude of the whole community. . . . [O]nly insofar as he takes the attitude of the organized social group to which he belongs toward the organized, co-operative social activity or set of such activities in which that group as such is engaged, does he develop a complete self or possess the sort of complete self he has developed. (pp. 154-155)

It is through the "me" and "the generalized other" that social control is exerted over the "I." It may also be the case, however, that the "I" and "me" can be in sync and become fused, as in certain religious or cooperative team experiences. This fusion can generate highly emotional experiences, a phenomenon Freud (1930/1962a) described as an "oceanic experience."

But Mead (1934) also tells us that social control is not total because of the unpredictability of the "I," and more important, from our social change perspective, that the individual's relationship with society is reciprocal. The "I" "is [the] one who reacts to [the] community and in his [sic] reaction . . . , changes it" (p. 196):

> if one puts up his [sic] side of the case, asserts himself over and against others and insists that they take a different attitude toward himself, then there is something important occurring that is not previously present in experience. (Mead, 1934, p. 196)

Conflicts can occur between different organized sets of attitudes or roles that make up an individual's self, between different individual selves, between subgroups within a society, between a subgroup within a society and the society as a whole, or between different societies. Finally Mead, sounding a bit like Marx, writes about the resolution of individual and social conflict:

> For it is their possession of minds or powers of thinking which enable human individuals to turn back critically, as it were, upon the organized social structure of the society of which they belong (and from their relations to which their minds are in the first instance derived), and to reorganize or reconstruct or modify that social structure to a greater or lesser degree, as the exigencies of social evolution from time to time require. Any such social reconstruction, if it is to be at all far reaching, presupposes a basis of common social interests shared by all the individual members of a given human society in which that reconstruction occurs; shared, that is, by all the individuals whose minds must participate in, or whose minds bring about, that reconstruction. (Mead, 1934, p. 308)

Let us now examine the clinical and social issues arising between two roles, Hispanic woman and lesbian, that, in part, may make up a self. We will use case material and expand the fine analysis from Carmen DeMonteflores' (1981) article "Conflicting Allegiances: Therapy Issues with Hispanic Lesbians." We choose this article because of its clarity, its thoughtfulness, its relevance, and because it is a good segue into the values, theory, and practice ideas we have developed. We are indebted to DeMonteflores and hope we do her ideas justice as we expand her conceptualization.

DeMonteflores correctly observes that the Hispanic community and the lesbian community are not monolithic and that individuals in these communities may vary a great deal as a result of their education, class background, religious affiliation, race, and so on. In the following, we will present many of DeMonteflores' generalizations about the attitudes, values, and beliefs of the Hispanic community and the lesbian community, recognizing that a particular Hispanic man or woman, and for our discussion a particular lesbian who may or may not be Hispanic, may vary a great deal from the generalizations we are about to make. Nevertheless, we believe that these generalizations will do the following:

- Highlight ideas about the development of two particular roles that can make up a self
- Highlight the potential conflicts that develop between parts of the self when a self is oriented to two reference groups that may have different values, norms, beliefs, ideas, and material aspects of culture and community that may be in conflict
- Help illuminate DeMonteflores' suggestions about clinical work
- Help to open a discussion about potential conflicts in our value base and how these conflicts may be addressed in practice

Growing up in the role of an Hispanic woman implies the socialization and internalization of a set of experiences, attitudes, norms, values, beliefs, and institutions, that is, a self related to the Hispanic community. DeMonteflores (1981) describes these attitudes in a selective way, focusing on how they would relate to the functioning of Hispanic lesbians. Specifically, she notes such things as the possibility of growing up in a traditional extended family, an emphasis on community life, experiences of racism that would make one wary of any primarily white subculture such as white lesbians, colorful dress, a set of negative attitudes and stigma related to homosexuality, and a description of "homosexuality as a white vice." While she does not focus on the lesbian community as extensively, she does note that politically oriented feminist lesbians place less value on monogamy, may see the nuclear family as "bankrupt and oppressive," value independence and autonomy, "coming out," and "political correctness," and may dress in a more "politically correct drab lesbian uniform." White lesbians, she adds, have also differentially internalized racist ideas from the larger society.

The Hispanic lesbian, whose self has internalized both the attitudes of her Hispanic birth culture and the lesbian community she has been socialized into as an adult, will surely have "conflicting allegiances." These conflicts are likely to develop and center on conflicting meanings and tensions related to the values of the two communities: closeness to family and community versus the wish for independence and autonomy, a reluctance about "coming out" versus a value supporting doing so, and how much attention to pay to dress and how colorful the dress should be. The Hispanic lesbian is also concerned about how much she can trust the white lesbian community.

In the clinical encounter, DeMonteflores (1981) suggests the need to ask and then listen to the self-definitions of Hispanic lesbians and engage the issues and conflicts that may emerge in the exploration of the multiple meanings of these self-definitions. She suggests that a white clinician, in particular, needs to be aware that an attempt to be politically correct may be patronizing to Hispanic lesbian clients. In addition, she cautions feminist therapists that their wish to be "liberal" and not to be seen as prejudiced may prevent them from appropriately challenging their Hispanic lesbian clients. "We must remember that individuals from minority groups also have psychodynamics like everybody else, and Hispanic lesbians are no exception" (p. 35). It is necessary to remember that workers also have psychodynamics and that attention must be paid to them as well.

Our value base has emphasized the self-determination of communities, groups, and individuals, economic and political justice, and a value related to the use of dialogical praxis as the primary tool for dealing with the first two values. These values have important implications for work with an Hispanic lesbian in an Hispanic community. On one hand, we would want to support a community's right to self-determination. But, in this case, the community's self-determination includes its stigmatization, if not oppression, of gay and lesbian individuals and groups in the community. Property rights, as we have demonstrated, can concretely infringe on the economic and political rights of others in the community. In some communities, property rights infringe on the majority of people. The sexual orientation of individuals in a community, on the other hand, may affect the sensibilities of members of a community but in no way can concretely affect their lives, politically and economically.

But sensibilities are important. Particularly in a multicultural society, dialogue between subgroups within a community and between communities can play a healing role. Dialogue can facilitate understanding, if not agreement, and acceptance of different aspects of another's life that does not infringe concretely on one's own life.

In our clinical work, we would hope to problematize what it means for a client to be an Hispanic lesbian, both within the Hispanic community and in the larger American society. Following Mead (1934), we presume a client's ability to "play" symbolic interactionist. Clients are able to be consciously self-reflective and understand how the attitudes of the two communities of which they are a part have been internalized and create conflict in their lives. Following DeMonteflores' injunction, we would also pay attention to the Hispanic lesbian's psychodynamics, her defenses, and other unconscious processes in an attempt to help her fully raise to consciousness both the internal and external dimensions of her conflicts. As part of the dialogue with a client, we understand that she may also be affected in concrete political and economic ways, both because of her status as an Hispanic woman and her status as a lesbian. These are concrete ways that affect her ability to be personally self-determining. This understanding would lead us as clinicians, assuming the client had an interest, to that part of dialogical praxis that includes action, such as political activity.

Political activity could take many forms here, including, but not limited to, developing an Hispanic lesbian support group, developing an Hispanic gay and lesbian support group, setting up a dialogue with members of the Hispanic community about the stigmatization of gays and lesbians, opening a dialogue with the larger lesbian community about racism, developing alliances between two oppressed communities, examining homophobic aspects of the worker's agency, developing therapeutic groups for gays and lesbians in the agency, dealing with social policies that affect a client and her communities, and so on. It is important to recognize the intimate connections between clinical work and social action issues and to deal with both concurrently.

We will end this chapter by describing the conflict our students have in taking this course after being socialized in much of the curriculum to maintain the dichotomy between clinical work and social action.

Some of our students, happily, find what we have to say refreshing. It hearkens back to their undergraduate days as social activists or to their experiences prior to coming to Smith. Some students, however, find our class an assault on the attitudes that respected teachers have socialized them to take and that they have come to share with peers. Their sense of self is mortified, to use Cooley's phrase, when we suggest that some of the attitudes, that is, values, norms, and beliefs, that they have learned may maintain oppression. The class uncovers a major contradiction in themselves that was rarely in their conscious awareness. Indeed, within the bulk of the curriculum it is easily denied. At best we hope that we help them resolve some of their contradictions through the practice skills we teach. When no resolution is possible, we attempt to help them recognize that they will have to live with some contradictions. In this case, we try to help them to come to terms with their own "funny walks."

Chapter 6

Critical Theory and Critical Practice

The philosophers have only interpreted the world, in various
ways; the point, however, is to change it.

Karl Marx, *Thesis on Feuerbach,* 1845

In this chapter we conclude the review and development of the
major aspects of our theoretical base. We will examine:

- the development of the Frankfurt School of critical theory and
  its relation to the theories of Marx, Freud, phenomenology,
  and symbolic interaction theory; and
- the influence of postmodern theory and particularly selected
  ideas of Michel Foucault.

Throughout this review, we will pay attention to the interaction
among values, theory, and practice. This review will set the stage
for our presentation of the critical theory and practice of Paulo
Freire that is developed throughout the rest of this book.

THE ROOTS OF CRITICAL THEORY

Felix Weil was a son of the wealthy Jewish businessman who
funded the Institute for Social Research at the University of Frankfurt in 1924. This institute became the center for the development of
critical theory. Weil was caught up in the socialist circles of Frankfurt (the German city with the highest percentage of Jews) and
studied with the Hungarian communist scholar Georg Lukacs. Carl

Grunberg, an academic Marxist, was the institute's first director. He committed the institute to social research grounded in Marxist ideology. Grunberg became ill in 1928 and was replaced in 1930 by Max Horkheimer. Horkheimer was a major, if not the central, charismatic figure in the development of critical theory. He was surrounded with colleagues and students such as Theodor Adorno, Erich Fromm, Herbert Marcuse, Walter Benjamin, and later Adorno's student, Jurgen Habermas (Wiggershaus, 1994). We will return to Max Horkheimer after examining two of the main influences on him and his fellow critical theorists, Karl Marx and Sigmund Freud.

KARL MARX

The young Karl Marx's observations and criticism of the political economy at the beginning of industrial capitalism in his *Economic and Philosophical Manuscripts* (1844/1978) powerfully affected the critical theorists of the Institute for Social Research. Essential for the development of our own integration of values and theory are the humanist values explicitly and implicitly embedded in this work. For example, Marx minces no words when he speaks of the degradation and "misery of the worker" that result from competition and "the accumulation of capital in a few hands" (1844/1978, p. 77).

Marx's discussion of alienation is particularly important. Workers, he wrote, have little if any control over their labor. They do not determine what products are produced or how products are produced and have no ownership of products after they are produced. Workers are alienated from what they produce and they themselves have become commodities in the process of production (Marx, 1844/1978):

> [W]ages and private property are identical: for wages, in which the product, the object of the labour, remunerates the labour itself, are just a necessary consequence of the alienation of labour. In the wage system the labour does not appear as the final aim but only as the servant of the wages. . . . [R]aising wages . . . would only mean a better payment of slaves and

would not give this human meaning and worth either to the worker or his [*sic*] labour. (p. 85)

Marx's values related to political and economic justice are clear when he calls for:

> [T]he positive abolition of private property and thus of human self-alienation and therefore the real reappropriation of the human essence by and for man [*sic*]. This is communism as the complete and conscious return of man conserving all the riches of previous development for himself as . . . social, i.e., human being[s]. . . . It is the genuine solution of the antagonism between man and nature and between man and man. (p. 89)

Expanding on Marx, Fromm (1961/1972) adds that the concept of alienation has its roots in Old Testament idolatry. "Idols are the work of man's [*sic*] own hands—they are things and man bows down and worships things; worships that which man created himself. In doing so he transforms himself into a thing" (Fromm, 1961/1972, p. 189). Then Fromm suggests:

> There is only one correction which history has made in Marx's concept of alienation; Marx believed that the working class was the most alienated class, hence that the emancipation from alienation would necessarily start with the liberation of the working class. Marx did not foresee the extent to which alienation was to become the fate of the vast majority of people, especially of the ever-increasing segment of the population which manipulate symbols and men [*sic*], rather than machines. . . . As far as consumption is concerned, there is no difference between the manual workers and the members of the bureaucracy. They all crave for things, new things to have and to use. (p. 195)

Marcuse (1966) makes a similar point in *One-Dimensional Man* that with the increased control of social welfare by for-profit organizations, social welfare workers should have little trouble recognizing the root and cause of their own current alienation. Nevertheless, Marx and later critical theorists hold out hopes for utopian solutions if private property can be abolished and true socialism, rather than a form of left fascism, can be put in place. For Fromm (1966) "Marx's concern was man [*sic*], and his aim was his liberation from the predomination of material interests . . ." (pp. 228-229).

SIGMUND FREUD

Paul Ricoeur (1970) links Freud and Marx into what he calls "the school of suspicion." Both question consciousness itself as not always being what it seems. But this questioning of consciousness has as its goal to open and illuminate the history of false consciousness in order to understand, criticize, and destroy its distortions (Roderick, 1986). The aim of this destruction is the development of a clearer consciousness that can be used by individuals to emancipate themselves from neurotic motivations. It hopes to free people for love and work that is not alienating. The self-reflective, free associative, critical, and interpretive processes of psychoanalysis are powerful methods that have been adopted by critical theorists to explore intrapersonal dynamics as well the dynamics of ideology and society that affect individuals and communities (Roderick, 1986). In the hands of the critical theorists, Freudian theory, while maintaining its influence as a dynamic psychology concerned with unconscious forces that motivate human behavior, feelings, and ideas, was transformed to take account of social and historical forces that affect individuals.

We agree with critical theorists' inclusion of the effects of social forces in understanding individual motivation. We do, however, question the attempt by some critical theorists/analysts such as Fromm (1966) to reduce or eliminate the relevance of the instincts and drives in human development. In addition, Marcuse's (1969) belief that the instincts themselves can be transformed (rather than in Freud's [1915/1963c] terms undergo vicissitudes) barring mutations seems to us wrong on its face. It appears motivated by Marcuse's wish, held by many critical theorists, for a utopian solution to ongoing human dilemmas, human limitations, and human lack of perfectibility. We disagree. The need for a dialogue and critique of the various levels and states of contradiction in society and ourselves is constant, even if/when a democratic socialist state can be established. Freud said that psychoanalysis is interminable; we would add that social analysis is also ongoing and interminable. Nevertheless, the explored life (Plato, 1992) has emancipatory and liberating potential that, while not utopian, and however ironic and even absurd, is worth living. As human beings, we can commit ourselves to engage in emancipatory self-reflection. It is then, like Camus's (1955) Sisyphus, whose "rock is his thing," that we can imagine ourselves happy.

Critical theorists recognized the need for Marx's theory to be supplemented by a psychology. Freudian theory and practice had the flexibility and more than enough of an emancipatory and critical edge to serve their purposes. For example, Fromm's (1966) concept of social character, which extends Freud's ideas about character, was useful. "The 'social character,' is that particular structure of psychic energy which is molded by any given society so as to be useful to the functioning of that society" (p. 231). Institutions of society mold social character. The family is particularly important in the first few years of life (Freud, 1905/1962b). But Fromm is clear that the family itself is shaped by social institutions and, most important, by economic institutions. As Peter Berger (1963) has noted, there are concentric rings of social control with the individual in the middle, the family and other primary groups in the next ring, and political and economic institutions in the outer ring, exerting pressures on the center. It is essential to recognize the internalization of aspects of the social world in an individual's unconscious. The social world then becomes part of the contents of an individual's unconscious (Fanon, 1967; Fromm, 1966). These unconscious ideas and ideologies shape, control, and repress what our students have labeled "dangerous thoughts." Dangerous thoughts are capable of raising consciousness about repressive and oppressive social systems. Dangerous thoughts raise awareness and create the possibility for change and emancipation.

MAX HORKHEIMER

As director of the Institute for Social Research in Germany and later, after escaping fascism, in the United States, Max Horkheimer played an important, if not central, role in the development of critical theory. His essay "Traditional and Critical Theory" (1937/ 1976) was seminal and laid a significant part of the foundation, however loose, for a set of ideas that has come to be known as critical theory. In this essay he contrasted his ideas with traditional theory. Many of the ideas for critical theory take their direction from the work of Marx and Engels while other ideas are grounded in the sociology, philosophy, and psychology of the early part of the twentieth century, for example, the sociology of Max Weber, the phenomenology of Edmund Husserl, and the psychology of Sigmund Freud.

Horkheimer (1937/1976), following Descartes, suggested that traditional theory and the model of mathematics start with a set of propositions from which deductions can be made in a relatively harmonious and seamless way. They can then be compared with observable facts. "If experience and theory contradict each other, one of the two must be re-examined" (p. 206). He notes the success of the traditional model of developing theory in the natural sciences and recognizes that most of the sciences, including the sociology of his time, have attempted to follow this model, that is, starting with the collection of facts so that these facts can be compared and formulated into theoretical concepts.

For Horkheimer, the problem with traditional theory is the assumption that objectivity is possible when observing the activities of men and women in their social world. In contrast, he points out that both the observer and the individuals taking part in social phenomena who are observed have a history that is rooted in society, and particularly, following Marx, in the economic arrangements of that society. For the critical theorist, the "facts" are socially produced.

An individual's perception of the world, that is, "facts" or ideas, through the senses is:

> socially preformed in two ways: through the historical character of the object perceived and through the historical character of the perceiving organ. Both are not simply natural; they are shaped by human activity, and yet the individual perceives himself [sic] passive in the act of perception. (Horkheimer, 1937/1976, p. 213)

It is essential that we recognize the subjective socially constructed element in all observations:

> As man [and woman] reflectively records reality, he [or she] separates and rejoins pieces of it, and concentrates on some particulars while failing to notice others. . . . Even where there is question of experiencing natural objects as such, their very naturalness is determined by contrast with the social world and, to that extent, depends on the latter. (pp. 214-215)

This theoretical view of reality is skeptical. Therefore, Horkheimer (1937/1976) posited the necessity of having a critical attitude "wholly distrustful of the rules of conduct with which the society as presently constituted provides each of its members" (p. 218). Those with a critical attitude are in constant tension with their society. They are distrustful of what is given as well as of what they perceive. Later, in Freire's practice, we see this as the need to problematize "facts and ideas." In the social phenomenologist's view of the world, we are required to look askance at the world taken-for-granted (Schutz, 1967).

Through this oppositional and dialectical view of the world, Horkheimer (1937/1976) hoped to "transcend the tension and abolish the opposition between the individual's purposefulness, spontaneity, and rationality, and those work-process relationships on which society is built" (p. 220). He observed the alienating effects of current economic organizational relationships and, without developing the "illusion of reaching for absolute knowledge," saw the possibility of critically examining and studying individuals in their economic relationships with concern for "men [*sic*] and all their potentialities" (p. 223). His hope was "to create a world which satisfies the needs and powers of men" (p. 224).

Critical theory is value based, not a neutral activity, and has no interest in the pretentious assumption of traditional theory to be value free, objective, and neutral. "Its goal is man's [*sic*] emancipation from slavery. . . . In radically analyzing present social conditions it became a critique of the economy" (Horkheimer, 1937/1976, pp. 223-224).

CRITICAL THEORY IN PRACTICE:
HERBERT MARCUSE'S REPRESSIVE TOLERANCE

Marcuse's (1965/1976) paper "Repressive Tolerance" is a fine example of critical theory in practice. His objective was to examine critically the idea and practice of tolerance in advanced industrial democracy. While acknowledging his preference for democratic tolerance over dictatorships, Marcuse also observed the repressive and oppressive aspects of tolerance as it is practiced under industrial capitalism. For example, he observes that while almost all speech is tolerated in Western democracies, the access to the distribution of speech, in and through the media, is not equal. The capitalist class owns and controls the major media and, without the need for a conspiracy, the members of that class protect their interests by printing and/or showing those programs which support their interests. General Electric, the owner of NBC, and Rupert Murdoch, the owner of Fox, have little interest in reporting on worker or consumer needs; that would challenge their hegemony. When they do report, it is in the interest of displaying their tolerance for free speech, and the reports are usually found on the back rather than the front pages. Like Horkheimer, Marcuse confronts the illusion of objectivity and neutrality as it is enacted in democratic tolerance. Specifically, he notes the homogenization and equal treatment of all information. Starvation and dying children in the Sudan, ethnic cleansing, "welfare reform," and the effects of managed care are given the same weight and delivered in the same monotone and with the same enthusiasm as "sexual scandal," aerobic exercises, a recipe for shrimp scampi, or the latest ads praising new or old products that may be necessary or just a new indulgence:

> A mentality is created for which right and wrong, true and false are pre-defined wherever they effect the vital interests of society. . . . [I]n a democracy with totalitarian organization, objectivity may fulfil [*sic*] a very different function, namely, to foster a mental attitude which tends to obliterate the difference between true and false, information and indoctrination, right and wrong. In fact, the decision between opposed opinions has been made before the presentation and discussion gets underway— made, not by a conspiracy or a sponsor or a publisher, not by any

dictatorship, but rather by the "normal course of events," which is the course of administered events, and by the mentality shaped in this course. (Marcuse, 1965/1976, pp. 310-311)

News talk shows advertising themselves as giving the opinions of left and right commentators present the viewer or listener with views spanning right wing Republicans to centrist Democrats. One looks hard to find a real socialist, let alone an articulate welfare recipient. An articulate recipient would describe in vivid detail the oppressive nature of workfare without adequate child care and what it means to choose between feeding herself and her children three adequate meals and paying the rent to avoid becoming homeless. The infighting between and capitulation of hospitals and social welfare organizations to insurance companies goes unreported. The alienation of doctors and social welfare workers who once could attempt to deliver their services in an honorable way is repressed. Too often now, welfare workers attempt to maintain jobs and income. They strive for a "good," if individualized, "self-actualized" life separate from politics, community involvement, and dialogue about the world in which they really exist.

Marcuse (1965/1976) challenges institutional violence that is tolerated, such as police violence in communities of color or the rates of infant mortality in minority communities that rival those of underdeveloped countries. "Non-violence," he suggests, "is normally not only preached to but exacted from the weak—it is a necessity rather than a virtue, and normally it does not seriously harm the case of the strong" (p. 315). Violence is not tolerated only when the "the oppressed rebel against the oppressors, the have-nots against the haves" (p. 316). In these cases, the owners of discourse speak of international terrorists who need to be rooted out, jailed, or killed, while, in social welfare organizations, advocates are labeled rabble rousers, leftists, unionists, and troublemakers who need to be rooted out, put in their place, and pilloried by being red-baited and fired.

Finally, Marcuse calls for the need to tolerate extralegal activities on the left and from oppressed groups when their nonviolent actions are unable to have an effect on the tolerated institutionally administered violence of democratic societies in which "false consciousness has become general consciousness":

[T]here is a "natural right" of resistance for oppressed and overpowered minorities to use extra-legal means if the legal ones have proved inadequate. Law and order are always and everywhere the law and order which protect the established hierarchy; it is nonsensical to invoke the absolute authority of this law and this order against those who suffer from it and struggle against it—not for personal advantage and revenge, but for their share of humanity. (1965/1976, p. 324)

Social welfare workers will need to make moral/value choices between a status quo that favors a variety of forms of repressive tolerance in their institutional work, or the values of political and economic justice, and self-determination that will ally them in dialogical praxis with the oppressed populations with whom they work. Social welfare workers who choose the critical approach need to come to terms with their outsider status, which is filled with tension and conflict, and lack of job security. In this way, they will be able to maintain their personal and professional values and begin to overcome the alienating contradictions in their work. The goal is a liberated and emancipated consciousness and connections with comrades in community.

MICHEL FOUCAULT AND POSTMODERN THEORY

Because of its current influence on social welfare theory and practice, as well as the contribution it can make to our thesis, we will examine, however selectively and critically, the work of Michel Foucault and postmodernism. Some of his most useful concepts are his discussions of the relationships among language, knowledge, discourse, and power. We also discuss his skepticism about individual emancipation, his ideas about local centers of power, and the need to understand and explore local contexts where political work can take place.

Central to Foucault is the concept of and the attempt to understand power. In his study and understanding of knowledge, language, and discourse, he emphasizes the implicit existence of power that dominates individuals. But Foucault also tells us that individuals cannot grasp either discourse or power to serve their own interests. "The individual is an effect of power . . . not its point of application" (quoted in S. T. Leonard, 1990, p. 69). Foucault's discourse, however critical, leaves little if any room for emancipatory alternative discourses (S. T. Leonard, 1990). For him, such discourses would themselves quickly become malicious and coercive.

S. T. Leonard (1990), however, attempted to rescue Foucault, perhaps from himself, by suggesting that Foucault left room in his later writing for individual subjectivity that could become conscious of a dominant discourse and substitute an alternative:

> If social agents, like Foucault himself, possess at least the potential for seeing previously unexamined and unarticulated presuppositions of language and practice as constraining where they need not be, then there must be some sense in which they can be the authors of their own actions. (p. 74)

Foucault's ideas related to the decentralization of power are important and parallel Freire's ideas about different localities needing to develop their own dialogue and praxis to free themselves from the particular oppressive situations they face. No longer is it useful to maintain the:

> illusion of "universal" solutions to situations of domination. . . . In other words, the power/knowledge grid was understood as producing relations of inequality, domination, and subordination differently in different localities, and different for different persons. Moreover, the localized character of power gives rise to localized, contextually specific forms of resistance. (S. T. Leonard, 1990, p. 75)

But Foucault's idea of liberation and freedom is, in the end, highly individual, related to the "body and pleasures" and has little to do with community. Even Leonard (1990), who is sympathetic to Foucault, notes this essential shortcoming in his work:

> The relation to oneself elides the difficult task of articulating the kind of collective action required to transform our relations with others in an emancipatory way. (S. T. Leonard, 1990, p. 79)

Even more devastating are critiques of Foucault and postmodernism that come from less sympathetic observers. For example, Prus

(1996) takes aim at postmodern skepticism and particularly the notion that "all forms of knowing (and presumably all forms of interpretation as well!)" are less than viable (p. 217) and "that no knowledge claims . . . should be privileged over any others" (p. 220).

The attraction of postmodernism, Prus sarcastically points out, is:

> [F]or those inclined to take viewpoints that might be deemed
> highly cynical, completely relativistic, persuasively despairing,
> intensely anti-scientific or anti-establishmentarian, or pointedly
> individualistic, postmodernism offers elements that are radical,
> fatalistic, absurd, and nihilistic in the extreme. (1996, p. 218)

Indeed, Prus suggests that postmodern academics have little trouble
privileging their own writing and ideas.

> If one were genuinely to acknowledge postmodern skepticism,
> there would be no incentive for anyone to do ethnographic re-
> search or gather any other sort of data or information about
> anything, since there is no privileged form of knowing (period!).
> (1996, p. 222)

More important, what Prus sees as missing from postmodernism is
the engagement of human beings with one another and with their
environment. Postmodernism is an intellectual retreat from politics:

> While some of us might want to offer a historical and material-
> istic explanation . . . for postmodernists the collapse of reality
> into its "representations" the disappearance of the line be-
> tween reality and fiction . . . actually is the reality of the late
> twentieth century. . . .

> Society has moved to the edge of a now flattened world, post-
> modernists claim, and the only fact that we can know with
> certainty is that we cannot understand what has moved us there
> or what lies down below, in the abyss. (Stabile, 1995, p. 90)

For our part, we value the more moderate skepticism and real
tensions involved in critical theory. However much it may be a
Sisyphean task, we value the goal of communal liberation and eman-

cipation that is embedded in critical theory. We are not interested in the extremes of individualistic sectarian (Freire, 1985) movements that see only their own oppression and but accept and even contribute to the oppression of others. Everything does not go for us! Our values are clear, and we strive for comradeship and solidarity with those who work to build a better society for all. We are concerned that, at its worst, postmodernism nihilistically may support the kind of repressive tolerance of the political economy of democratic industrial capitalism that Marcuse so eloquently challenged.

Chapter 7

The Contradictions in Clinical Work

In Chapter 1, we introduced the concept of contradiction and suggested its centrality in bridging the gap between clinical work and social action. In this context, contradictions are the inconsistencies, discrepancies, antagonisms, or lack of truth (Guralnick, 1970) between what workers, agencies, professions, and other social institutions profess to be about, their values and mission statements, and the behaviors and policies they enact in their work with clients.

For Marx and Engels (1970), the essential contradictions are economic and are played out in class antagonisms and class conflicts within the political economy. Any examination of practice in the human services needs to take account of this level of contradiction. Critical theorists, however (Findlay, 1978; Marcuse, 1965/1976, 1966, 1969), must also pay attention to the psychological, technological, bureaucratic, and other aspects of practice that create and shape contradictions. These interests and forces may overlap, complement, exclude, or be mutually antagonistic. They determine the meanings of contradictions and develop the compromises that manifest and express the conflicts within contradictions. However, political, economic, emotional, and other interests are also at play that inhibit workers and organizations from examining, engaging, and attempting to resolve contradictions. For us, it is the reflective process inherent in the problematization of clinical work that allows the discovery of both the contradictions that play out in practice and the political, economic, interpersonal, and individual interests and forces that create the contradictions in the clinical encounter.

The primary direction of power and influence shaping behavior, as well as individual and collective social action, is from the political economy to levels below it. Social change, however, can arise from the level of clinical work, the level at which workers meet clients, to affect higher levels. It is from the level of clinical work that the dialogical praxis that guides our work begins to move toward social action. Clinicians must generally deal with and work on their own contradictions before engaging other contradictions at other levels, that is, within the agency, the profession, professional education, and the political economy. Exploration at the clinical level will, however, often illuminate other issues that require engagement. For example, an Anglo worker might value working with an Hispanic client in the client's own language. The worker, however, does not speak Spanish. The problematization and exploration of this contradiction at the clinical level could open contradictions in an agency that had no bilingual workers and no classes in Spanish, even as the agency's mission statement purports to promote cultural sensitivity and to serve a diverse clientele.

What follows are examples and beginning analyses of contradictions that can be observed in clinical work. Given the many determinants of a contradiction, we expect that many levels of contradictions will be present simultaneously. We will make these different levels explicit even as we focus on each level individually. We begin with contradictions at the level of the worker.

CONTRADICTIONS IN CLINICAL WORK AT THE LEVEL OF THE WORKER

Consciously and unconsciously, human service workers often act as if there were no contradictions in their work with the people they serve. It would be most gratifying and uncomplicated for progressive workers to see their sole motivation for entering the human service professions as a moral imperative based in values such as the essential worth of every human being and a wish to help the poor and oppressed. In fact, the range and quality of motivations are complex and the meanings that shape these motivations are often contradictory. Some are relatively benign, though not without problems, while others can be quite malignant. To paraphrase and extend Freire (1989a), a psychoanalysis of the professions might reveal a "false generosity" based on guilt or a wish to buy peace rather than a willingness to engage in authentic dialogue.

For example, workers are often in a position to "generously," if paternalistically, dole out benefits, goods, services, and cash to clients from whom they, the workers, benefit. As part of their professional role, workers have higher status, power, and privilege than almost all their clients. In addition, the client is expected to be grateful in this inequitable transaction. The client should not show anger and must give up any wish to struggle against the system that pays, and is represented by, the worker. A worker's experience of doing good works should not be threatened. A client on welfare described her situation this way:

> I'm always playing a role when I go to the Welfare Department. It's like going on a date. I think about what I'm going to wear and how I'm going to act and what I need to do to please them with the least amount of honesty about who I really am. (Withorn, 1996, p. 278)

Supplying or advocating for needed benefits assuages whatever guilt the worker may have about the client's situation and buys peace into the bargain. It subjugates clients, knowledge, experience, and feelings. The black feminist thinker Patricia Hill Collins (1991) writes that subjugating knowledge "makes it easier for dominant groups to rule because the seeming absence of an independent consciousness in the oppressed can be taken to mean that subordinate groups willingly collaborate in their own victimization" (p. 5). This is a type of cultural invasion in which workers "impose their own view of the world upon those they invade and inhibit the creativity of the invaded by curbing their expression" (Freire, 1989a, p. 150).

Problematizing the "generosity" of workers within the clinical encounter opens the possibility of workers and the people they serve becoming aware of the contradictions in practice and the relationship workers and the people they serve have to those in power. "Those [workers] who make this discovery face a difficult alternative: To renounce invasion would mean ending their dual status as dominated and dominators" (Freire, 1989a, p. 154). Many workers, however, are fearful of this new consciousness. They are unwilling to give up their professional identities and status. Through a series of evasions, they choose to rationalize the contradictions of their position, attack those who raise their consciousness about their contradictions, and blame their clients, who express their own new and clearer view of their world, as ungrateful and unworthy.

The experience of one of the authors, happily with a good ending, will illustrate the contradictions and dilemmas faced by even the most well intentioned workers. It is an example of how one can contribute to oppression even as one fights it.

Jerry Sachs had, for several years, been a coleader of a group of homeless people with a formerly homeless woman and a young paraprofessional man. At one point, in his professional "wisdom," or, on clearer reflection, professional arrogance, elitism, possible sexism, and classism, he thought that he, rather than his female coleader, should attend an important meeting related to homelessness in the community. In the name of doing what he, "an expert," thought best for an oppressed group, he attempted to subjugate the knowledge and voice his female coleader had acquired living and surviving on the street for more than a year. He even had "explanations," read rationalizations, for his behavior that included words such as "her transference," "her projective identification," "her lack of boundaries," "her subjectivity," and so forth. Sachs did know better than to say these words out loud.

Blessedly, his coleader would have none of it and, with the support of the young paraprofessional, confronted Sachs, opening Sachs' contradictions and oppressiveness. Having the contradiction problematized, Sachs was able to acknowledge and reflect on it. With his coleaders, he was able to understand it as a way to protect his status, power, and privilege, even as he valued cooperation and equality between workers.

Playfully, when he got out of hand after this, his coleaders gently and humorously tweaked him by referring to him as Dr. Sachs rather than as Jerry. Usually he got the message. At times, through dialogue with his coleaders, they found together that their tweaking was misplaced. Sachs' co-workers recognized the importance of problematizing their own actions and the need to maintain the integrity of everyone's voice, even a professional's.

It is necessary to understand deeply and examine critically how power, status, and privilege are at stake when, consciously and unconsciously, workers, in contradiction to their own stated values, divide and label the people they work with into good cases and bad cases, the worthy and unworthy poor, the resistant cases and well-motivated cases. This labeling is an act of bad faith and usually involves the worker's own insecure sense of goodness, worthiness, and motivation. To give up status, privilege, and power is a psychological loss that may also involve material losses such as buying a home or a second home, taking a vacation of choice or a second vacation, and eating out, eating well, or not eating at all.

A WORD ABOUT COUNTERTRANSFERENCE AND CONTRADICTIONS

In our classes and workshops, some participants have difficulty differentiating between countertransference and contradictions. In the simplest terms, countertransference is the transference of a worker toward the people he or she serves. Though "effected . . . by conscious ideas and expectations, [they are also effected] by those [ideas and expectations] that are under repression, or unconscious" (Freud, 1912/ 1963b, p. 107). They are a cliché or stereotype developed from experiences in childhood "which perpetually reproduces itself as time goes on" (pp. 105-106). They can be recognized by their "excess, in both character and degree, over what is rational and justifiable" (p. 107). For example, a worker may have an issue with passivity or anger or sexuality. The content of these issues, a product of his or her particular developmental history as a child, may create difficulties for this worker when engaging with people on issues of advocacy, child abuse, race, class, homophobia, gender, and so on.

Countertransference, however, may or may not create a contradiction, that is, a conflict between a worker's personal or professional values and his or her actions with clients in the clinical work. For example, a worker may have a countertransferential identification with a client's oppressor or a countertransferential identification with the client as an oppressed person. In the first case, the worker's countertransference would influence his or her willingness to side with oppressive actions against the client. In the second case, the worker's countertransference would influence his or her to side with the client against oppressive action. In this example, the dynamics of one countertransference would reinforce a worker's professional value to fight oppression and create a contradiction with the dynamics of the other countertransference. Indeed, we can even imagine a worker's countertransference working against his or her own class interest. What is important to recognize is that contradictions based in countertransference will need to be worked through (Freud, 1914/1963e), in the psychological sense, before they may be able to be resolved consciously at a political level.

CONTRADICTIONS IN AGENCIES

Public and private social welfare agencies are bureaucratic organizations that have goals and functions related to missions and objectives defined by legislation and/or contributors who fund them. To implement the mission of an agency, an organization develops policies, structures, and procedures that serve to control how people connected with the agency will behave:

> Much of the power of the organization over its workers [and clients] is invisible and operates through the standard operating procedures. The agency, in effect, controls the decision-making processes of its workers [and clients] by constraining the type of information they will process, by limiting the range of alternatives available to them, and by specifying the decision rules for choosing among alternatives. (Hasenfeld, 1987, p. 471)

In some organizations there may be few contradictions between the progressive values we have espoused, progressive values developed by professional associations, and the goals, functions, and objectives derived from an organization's mission statements. Grassroots organizations such as the American Indian Movement, a welfare rights organization, or self-help groups such as the Alliance for the Mentally Ill sometimes hire professional workers as consultants. These workers supply expertise, remain accountable to the communities they serve and, consequently, have few contradictions. But, as Freire suggests, both workers and community people are likely to have their feet in both progressive and oppressive worlds when they access funds from government or foundations that have their own agendas and are removed from the communities that are served.

Many organizations, however, contradict the progressive values of workers and/or progressive professional values. This contradiction happens most often in control organizations such as prisons or mental hospitals whose functions are antithetical to dialogical praxis and the self-determination of the people who are housed in them. Ohlin, Piven, and Pappenfort (1956) described the levels of co-optation that workers undergo, and Garfinkle (1956) and Goffman (1961) described the degradation ceremonies and betrayal funnels developed by prisons and mental hospitals.

For example, as an MSW student, one of the authors was told by a recent graduate that he needed to be aware of the control functions of the halfway house for prisoners that was going to be his field placement. Within six months, however, the author learned that his would-be mentor was now a prison system employee. When a prisoner escaped, the mentor was told to take a gun to participate in the search for the convict, and he agreed. Too often, being co-opted by an agency is easier for workers than living and struggling with the contradictions that agencies pose.

But even "benign" organizations whose missions are to serve clients and promote self-determination often find that their original goals are displaced by new goals (Merton, 1940) that create contradictions. These new goals are often related to an agency's survival and the smooth functioning of the organization's administration and workers. This is true even when it is at the expense of the people the organization is set up to serve. A child welfare worker was told by her supervisor to "cool out" an angry mother who was going to take her complaints to the Bureau of Child Welfare (Sachs, 1987). Though most mental health agencies would say they value understanding the meanings of expressed emotions, few easily tolerate the expression of anger or complaints against the agency. Agencies regularly provide poor quality care or terminate services to angry and complaining clients.

With the advent of managed care, agencies that valued and prided themselves on long-term work with clients now demand that workers move clients in and out of their system quickly. They follow the parameters set by insurers and their own financial needs rather than meeting the needs of the people in communities they serve. Legal services lawyers who have been involved in case advocacy with clients on welfare have found that their agency's policies prohibit them from bringing these clients together in groups.

Some organizations are in contradiction to their own stated missions. A child welfare agency's mission statement read that children in its care will be placed in the most "appropriate setting." Nevertheless, the agency had a funding-driven policy barring the transfer of children outside of the agency structure.

Given the contradictions that are rooted in an agency's policies, structure and functions, workers are forced to compromise their personal and professional values and clients suffer from oppressive conditions. Long ago, Bertha Capen Reynolds (1982, p. 107) suggested, in clear dialogical fashion, a first step out of this trap: "The case worker might well talk out with the clients the fact that these decisions [contradictions] are governed by principles which bind him [sic] no less than the client and are the reality which they both must face." This type of dialogue, "focusing on conflict, constraints, contradictions, and the power of the status quo" (Findlay, 1978, p. 62), however, has its problems for progressive workers particularly in a "society [or an agency] that values consensus, agreement and going along" (Findlay, 1978, p. 62). The outcome for social welfare workers who adopt a progressive set of values and a dialogical method would, therefore, include dismay, conflict with fellow workers and administrators, living with contradictions, and little job security (Findlay, 1978). Fortunately, there is what we have called "wiggle room" in almost all situations that allows progressive workers to operate against the grain and work with hope toward greater dialogue and freedom for themselves and the people they serve. Ira Shor (1996, p. 3), integrated similar ideas this way:

> Freire [1994] described "limit acts" which push against the borders of what's possible, to test what is feasible. His notion of "untested feasibility" was formulated differently by Michel Foucault (1980), who wrote that "there is indeed always something in the social body, in classes in groups and individuals themselves which in some sense escapes relations of power, something which is by no means more or less docile or reactive primal matter, but rather a centrifugal movement, an inverse energy, a discharge" (p. 138). Put another way, Raymond Williams (1977) emphatically argued that "*no mode of production therefore no dominant social order and therefore no domi-*

nant culture ever in reality includes or exhausts all human practice, human energy, and human intention." (italics in the original)

CONTRADICTIONS IN THE PROFESSIONAL ROLE

The profession of social work has played major roles in the history of social welfare. These roles have often been progressive, sometimes oppressive, but almost always contradictory. Social work is also the profession the authors inhabit and with which they are most familiar. We will therefore look to social work as our primary example for examining contradictions in the social welfare professions.

Social work has a long and honorable history bringing attention to the needs of oppressed people. There was a clear lapse in the priorities of the previous *NASW Code of Ethics* (Sachs, 1990) for issues of social justice. The current code of the National Association of Social Workers, adopted in 1997, however, includes and emphasizes values and goals such as:

- Social workers' primary goal is to help people in need and to address social problems
- A focus on social justice
- Social workers challenge social injustice
- Cultural competence and social diversity
- Self-determination

It is ironic, therefore, that as social work has successfully professionalized and "legitimated" itself through licensure, laws covering third party payments, and private practice that its historical mission to serve poor and oppressed people has wavered:

Much of the basis for this lies in the very nature of professions under capitalism. In exchange for social status, monopoly over certain useful functions, the ability to police themselves and have a measure of self-determination over the nature and conditions of their work, society demands conformity and mainstream ideology. The more prestigious the profession, the more this holds true. In essence, society confers privilege for a price and the price is not rocking the boat. While social work has not achieved the status and power of older and more male-dominated professions, the professionalization of caring has been accompanied by a decrease in the degree to which that caring has been enacted in a politically aware context. Professionalization of social work has led to a deification of technique over social justice; a concern for protecting professional status even at the cost of assigning client concerns a lower priority. (Newdom, 1996, p. 1)

In addition, becoming a full profession has separated master's degree social workers from paraprofessional social welfare workers at different levels of education, training, and years of experience. Inclusion and connection with other workers has given way to exclusiveness and monopoly over practice. This monopoly extends social work's control over other workers and clients. Ironically, these practices open social work to the criticism it leveled at professional medical people who were and still are seen as oppressing lower status professional social workers.

Closely tied to the professionalization of human services, and particularly the professionalization of social work, is the political and economic inequality that come with increased status and privilege. This status differential creates disengagement from clients and is a major contradiction for professional workers. To deal with this contradiction, professional social workers claim the need for neutrality and objectivity. But the claim of neutrality, as Freire (1985) observes, "does not constitute neutrality; quite the contrary, it helps maintain the status quo" (p. 39). Social workers are constantly making choices between reactionary and progressive options. To see an issue as a social problem or an individual deficit, to continue or discontinue work with an angry confrontational client, to engage in dialogue or exert control over paraprofessional workers and clients, to problematize the world or give in to the status quo, to act as an agent of social control or an agent of change, and to bear witness or be silent are some of the political choices social workers make every day.

What is needed is to problematize the situation and the actions of social workers. We need to reflect deeply and critically with each other and the people we serve in order to bear witness for political and economic justice. Social welfare workers should recognize and struggle with the contradictions that professionalism brings with it. We must move away from professionalism and toward a more egalitarian relationship with the people who are served by us. The place to begin this critical reflection and engagement is in clinical practice.

CONTRADICTIONS IN SOCIAL WORK EDUCATION

As we noted in Chapter 1, teaching from a Freirian perspective in a university-based human services program represents another contradiction (Leonard, 1993). In the university, a Freirian approach invariably will produce tensions between "traditional" pedagogy which imparts content and Freirian pedagogy in which content emerges through a dialogical praxis. There are also tensions between the school's and the students' expectations of the professor role and the professor being a participant in a process of dialogical learning. Another tension is between the professor and students meeting in the world as equal Subjects and the expectation that the professor will judge and evaluate, i.e., objectify the work of students. Chapters 9 to 14 will be devoted to different aspects of teaching and our experience as faculty. The contradictions in teaching will be part of those discussions.

CONTRADICTIONS IN THE POLITICAL ECONOMY

The contradictions in social welfare arising from the political economy are powerful and profound. The political economy affects all levels of social relations within social welfare institution, that is, agencies, the professions, the individual worker, and the client more powerfully and consequentially than they can affect the political economy. The self-interested profit motive of capitalism in the United States leaves little room for political and economic justice, self-determination of communities, or dialogical praxis unless they too can somehow be made to turn a profit. To the extent that it can, industry will use government, as it did in the 1981 air traffic controllers' strike, to bust unions and send a message to workers that the propertied class runs the economy and controls their survival. To the extent that social welfare agencies can be made to cooperate in the capitalists' project, however much it may be contradictory to the mission of these agencies and its workers, it will be done.

The role of social welfare organizations in the Hormel strike (1985-1986) in Minnesota illustrate this principle. Rachleff (1993) reported that the hope of the strikers was that the Hormel Foundation, which controlled 46 percent of Hormel stock and received tax breaks from the state for serving the interests of the local community, would come to their aid. In fact the foundation

> became a tool in the hands of corporate management to control the behavior of local charitable organizations—the Mower County Mental Health Clinic, St. Olaf Hospital and the Salvation Army. . . . The Foundation was a major donor to most of these organizations, and representatives of corporate management sat on their boards.

> Hormel's tentacles reached deeply into these community institutions and provided them with powerful tools to turn against the strikers. The Mower County Mental Health Clinic decried the strike as a source of stress in the community and its director launched a virtual back to work campaign. . . . St. Olaf Hospital refused to release any information on injuries in the Hormel plant to the media. The Mower County Food Shelf initially turned away strikers' families who sought assistance. . . . Even the local churches refrained from criticizing Hormel [and some] were willing to house National Guardsmen sent [to break] picket lines. (Rachleff, 1993, pp. 76-77)

Human service workers are members of what Barbara and John Ehrenreich (1979) have called the professional managerial class (PMC). Situated between owners of property and the people they serve in social welfare agencies, the PMC have their own interests, which often conflict with the values of the power elite and the needs of the people they serve. Upper-class elites control the boards, shape the policies, and approve the programs PMC technocrats are expected to implement. It is these elites who define the policies of the institutions in which they work. The PMC nevertheless have a value system that reflects service to poor, oppressed, and disenfranchised populations. It is this value system, rooted in religious and humanistic beliefs, that sets the stage for the contradictions in which the PMC is caught. We see this clearly in the example of the Hormel strike.

The contradictions are clear when social workers profess dedication to clients and community and then act as oppressors serving the interests of the propertied class that control the institutions that pay their salaries. When clients then attack agencies and workers, no one should be surprised by their attack.

Professionals and professions suffer from false consciousness, not recognizing that they are workers rather than owners of property, or that when they are owners it is of small shops, for example, private practice, and not large corporations. For example, social workers during the 1980s and early 1990s moved ever closer to full professionalization and made a dramatic entry into private practice. Recently, however, the real capitalists arrived in the form of large insurance companies, managed care corporations, and HMOs, leading to the consolidation of hospitals and social welfare agencies. Social workers, as well as other health professionals, find that they have ever less control over their work (Fabricant and Burghardt, 1992). It is the corporate insurers that increasingly own and control a professional's work. Students and older workers talk more and more of the alienation they experience as they are forced by managed care and their agencies to terminate clients prematurely. "With this division of labour, in which all these contradictions are implicit. . . . This latent slavery is . . . property . . . the power of disposing of the labour-power of others" (Marx and Engels, 1970, pp. 52-53). Whether social welfare workers become politically conscious of the narrow self-interests they have pursued and join with other workers to eliminate the alienation they suffer from is yet to be seen.

THE INTENSITY OF CONTRADICTIONS

Contradictions vary in intensity to the extent that the forces that make up the contradiction are meaningful and valued. Fee policies at mental health clinics often create high-intensity contradiction for workers. Agency administrations demand that workers see only those clients who pay their fees as arranged. Often, workers are labeled as being in "countertransference" if they question policies negatively affecting clients. Workers also fear being sanctioned when they go against agency policies.

A worker's practice with a thirteen-year-old African-American girl illustrates how a worker's values can clash with a policy on fees. The client had done well in treatment and gave the worker a good deal of satisfaction. She had "high therapeutic worth" (Sachs, 1989). The client, however, came without her fee on the first session after intermitting treatment for two months. She had stopped treatment in order to pay off fees she had in arrears. The contradiction was clear and well stated by the worker:

> A classic example is that issue with that other client. You know, I really found myself wanting to give her the benefit of the doubt, really wanting to get this kid back in treatment 'cause the kid needed it, and I realized that I was responding on different levels, that administratively I realized that I was going to be up the creek when this client was back in with fee arrears and that things haven't been resolved after clinically, supposedly, I had dealt with it and worked it out with the client. On another level, kind of feeling a little angry at the client for putting me in this position. . . .
>
> I was really going to have to account for it. . . . I mean anybody looking in on it, . . . whether their . . . perspective was administrative [or clinical] so that the two don't always mesh and yet we act as if they do here. That there's a real feeling that, you know, that what makes good clinical sense, you know, is what administratively makes sense too, and sometimes it doesn't. And it gets me in a bind or whatever.

We conclude by suggesting that the intensity of a contradiction will play a role in determining the degree to which a worker is likely to feel stress, tension, anxiety, and alienation on the job. As a measure of job satisfaction, these feelings will no doubt affect a client's therapeutic worth and the treatment he or she receives.

Chapter 8

Action and Reflection in Work with a Group of Homeless People

Social workers who see themselves as social activists have fewer professional and bureaucratic supports for their activities than they did at any time since the 1960s. Part of the reason is the systematic dismantling of the gains made during the War on Poverty since the Nixon administration. Another, perhaps more important, reason is the success social work has had in professionalizing, that is, gaining licensure, increasing the opportunities for private practice, and becoming eligible for third-party payments (Sachs, 1990).

Ironically, as social work professionalized, it simultaneously began to give up its commitment to social activism, social justice and work with oppressed groups (Sachs, 1990). As the profession and individual social workers have gained status, social work has become engaged, though not yet wedded, to the more conservative trends in the political economy (Cloward and Piven, 1976; Newdom, 1996).

Despite this trend, social work still remains one of the few professions with a rich history of social activism at both the clinical and policy level and selectively continues to promote this tradition. Affordable housing and homelessness are two related issues in which the profession and individual workers continue the historic tradition of social action.

Work related to these issues provides the backdrop for this chapter. Attention will be directed to work with a group of homeless

Another version of this chapter appeared in the journal *Social Work with Groups.* Sachs, J. (1991), Volume 14, pp. 187-202, under the title "Action and Reflection in Work with a Group of Homeless People."

people in a rural New England town of 18,000. This chapter is organized around five phases or issues in the group's development:

1. The decision to work with the homeless
2. The engagement process
3. The first action
4. Dealing with identification with the oppressor
5. The last action

The author, Sachs, would note that this is a personal narrative and is therefore filled with distortions and omissions. It is, however, just these distortions which may reveal, for better and worse, the contradictions and ambivalence in values, beliefs, biases, countertransferences, and theory assumptions (real and imagined), that precipitate a worker's action.

Insofar as outside observers, or workers themselves, can take account of the historic forces that make up the work, they can better understand the meanings of a worker's motivations and behavior (Schutz, 1967). For example, when Sachs was studying for his Bar Mitzvah, he read a story of how a great rabbi was struck with leprosy when he turned away from a calf being taken to slaughter. Years later, the story continued, the rabbi was cured when he fed milk to some orphaned kittens. Indeed, Sachs' stock answer, when asked how he came to get involved in social and political issues, is "to avoid leprosy." A trained analyst, he recognized a deep truth. The unconscious does not lie, however much it is filled with conflict, ambivalence, ambiguity, and mystery.

Both Freudians and Marxists understand the importance of consciousness raising. They are both aware of the freeing effect of understanding the motivations of one's actions through reflection:

> . . . a revolution is achieved with neither verbalism nor activism, but rather with praxis, that is, with reflection and action directed at the structures to be transformed. The revolutionary effort to transform these structures radically cannot designate its leaders as its thinkers and the oppressed as mere doers. (Freire, 1989a, p. 120)

What Freire makes clear is that the structure that is often in great need of transformation is the mind and thinking of the leader. This is particularly important when one works with a group whose class interests, not to mention values, history, culture, race, gender, sexual orientation, or lifestyle are different than one's own. Where one gains materially, however indirectly, from those differences, or when one's employment as a worker derives from the very existence of the social problem, self-awareness is critical. Otherwise,

> the leaders [will] treat the oppressed as mere activists to be denied the opportunity of reflection and allowed merely the illusion of acting, whereas in fact they would continue to be manipulated and in this case by the presumed foes of manipulation. (Freire, 1989a, p. 120)

THE DECISION TO WORK WITH THE HOMELESS

Between 1988 and 1989, the Northeastern Housing Organization (NHO), a grassroots membership organization made up of tenants, homeowners, and housing advocates, put a rent control by-law proposal before the town council of Mapleton. The bylaw was designed to control the 18 to 20 percent per year average rise in rent that had taken place in the town during the previous five years. This rise in rents was, no doubt, connected to the 32 percent increase in requests for emergency shelter over the previous year.

In 1989, after much debate, the town council voted to put the rent control bylaw up for a referendum. The selectboard and town council (both made up heavily of real estate interests) and the local newspaper came out against the proposal. The campaign against the bylaw was, at times, vicious. It included red-baiting, harassing phone calls to women in leadership, misinformation, and less-than-subtle intimidation of some tenants.

NHO consolidated its leadership in a six-person steering committee, which included the author. The group's mailing list grew to over 150. Debates about the bylaw proposal were held on the local radio and at public forums. As a result, consciousness about homelessness and the need for affordable housing was raised in the town. Though the by-law was defeated almost 2-1, it was the largest turnout in an off-year election in the town's history. It made NHO a force to be taken seriously.

After the referendum, the core group of NHO licked its wounds, hired a new VISTA worker (the only paid staff), and rested. At their September meeting they shared summer experiences, assessed the gains and losses from the rent control campaign, and explored ideas about how they might work with low-income and homeless people.

The group did not have to look far. Some of its members and the new VISTA worker had themselves been homeless. In October, the newspaper reported people living in tents in the woods, and funds for a year-round emergency shelter had been denied.

Sachs had worked with homeless groups in single-room occupancy housing (SRO) in New York City and just finished reading Paulo Freire's *Pedagogy of the Oppressed*. He wondered whether Freire's dialogical principles could be applied to work with a group of homeless people in rural New England:

> The dialogical theory of action does not involve a Subject, who dominates by virtue of conquest, and a dominated object. Instead there are Subjects who meet to name the world in order to transform it. If at a certain historical moment the oppressed . . . are unable to fulfill their vocation as Subjects, the posing of their very oppression as a problem (which always involves some sort of action) will help them achieve this vocation.

> . . . in the dialogical task . . . leaders—in spite of their important, fundamental and indispensable role—do not own the people and have no right to steer the people blindly toward their salvation. . . . Dialogue does not impose, does not manipulate, does not domesticate, does not "sloganize."

> . . . cooperation leads dialogical Subjects to focus their attention on the reality which mediates them and which—posed as a problem—challenges them. (Freire, 1989a, pp. 167-168)

At the October meeting of the NHO, there was a consensus to try to organize a group for homeless people. Three people from NHO would work together: Ellen, a formerly homeless woman; Steve, a young paraprofessional who had previously been a VISTA worker in a food and clothing distribution program in town; and Sachs. In addition, Deb, the new VISTA worker, had recently been homeless and knew the network of services for homeless people.

Contradiction

Sachs is no revolutionary. At best and at times he has been a radical and at worst, a liberal. He owns his own home, is relatively privileged, and knows he would gain professionally from participating in the group. On the other hand, he would be involved even if there was no professional gain since he worries about getting leprosy. He also has a history of using his power and privilege to advocate and intervene on the side of social justice.

Practice Principles

Social workers committed to reflecting on their actions do well to have other activists around. The more diverse the backgrounds of these activists the better. Everyone is kept honest by the different perspectives, and the possibility for "ego tripping" is kept to a minimum. In addition, the time commitment of the most disciplined volunteers, or even full-time workers, is limited. It is essential to have backup. There is also a need to share feelings and ideas, ventilate frustrations, and be connected.

In the leadership group, for example, there was some initial deference to the author as the initiator of the idea to engage homeless people and the person with the most group leadership experience. The other two leaders, however, quickly began to play crucial roles in the process. For example, before the group began, Ellen was quick to let Sachs know that, for all his book learning, "social workers can really be terrible and don't understand the needs of homeless people . . . you have to be there," as she had been. In addition, Steve and Deb knew the social service system and how to work it. This unfamiliar territory to the "Doctor," the name Steve affectionately called Sachs when he wanted to tweak him and bring him down to earth.

Clinical Work

It did not escape the author that Ellen's anger had some transferential elements, that is, was excessive and too repetitive (Freud,

1912/1963b). Though he often acknowledged the truth of many of her feelings about the destructive role of social workers with disenfranchised people, he also took the opportunity, as their relationship developed, to ask why she felt a need to deal with him as she did. Though Sachs was a social worker who made many mistakes, he was also far from the "rotten workers" she described from her past.

On the other hand, transference always has a hook in reality. On reflection, Sachs had treated Ellen condescendingly. For example, he thought it more important that he rather than she attend an important meeting. She was angry and talked about it with Steve, who suggested she call Sachs. She did and Sachs apologized. Ellen forgave him and has since been able to see him more as an individual than a "social worker."

THE ENGAGEMENT PROCESS

The place to find large groups of low-income and homeless people in Mapleton is at the community meals program in one of the local churches. Deb, the VISTA worker, was asked to make contact with the head of the meals program and determine if she would introduce us to homeless people. The head of the program agreed and that week introduced us to two homeless men. The first question the men asked us was "What do you want?!" The question was anticipated. We explained who we were. We said we were not sure we could be helpful but thought it worthwhile to see if we could. We hoped to meet with them and talk about what their concerns were and what they wanted. The fact that Ellen could say she had been homeless was important and gave us some credibility. They also felt good that we were all volunteers and did not work for a social agency.

When we felt there was the beginning of a relationship, we asked whether they would be willing to meet with us after the meal the following week and if other homeless people they knew might be interested. They said "sure" but told us condescendingly that we really did not understand. If the group ran late, they would get to their tent in the woods when it was "too late." We quickly guaranteed transportation "home" to anyone who came to the group. Some of their skepticism disappeared. We then drove them, on a drizzly thirty-five-degree night, to the edge of a secluded wood, where they disappeared. Sachs commented to his co-activists how strange it was to see them disappear. We all wondered how they would fare as the weather moved toward freezing conditions.

The following week, three homeless men and two homeless women attended our meeting. Each told his or her story and we were somewhat helpful in directing them to services that might be useful to them. We gave them names of people to contact at Legal Services and the local community action office. We also gave them our phone numbers and promised to follow up if there were any problems.

The group members also told us of the general needs of homeless people. We were learning. We helped them and the group agreed to meet again. By the third week, we were twelve and by the fourth week, fifteen.

Contradictions

When we took the men home to the woods the second week, it was thirty degrees and snowing. After we dropped them off, we talked about the contradictions of going home to our warm houses. We were also angry at some of the local politicians who talked about opening the Town Hall for emergency shelter and then re-neged.

Though some emergency shelter money had been raised to fund the homeless shelter program, the shelter itself was not going to be opened for two weeks. The previous year a homeless person had frozen to death on the railroad tracks and we were not willing to take homeless people into our own homes (another contradiction), however much each of us thought about doing so. Sachs knew it was easier to advocate and give money for food than to deal with what it would mean to have a relatively unknown homeless person share a roof with him, his wife, and his young daughter.

PRACTICE PRINCIPLES

In his discussion of cultural invasion, Freire (1989a) points out that:

. . . professionals (because of their very fear of freedom . . .) repeat the rigid patterns in which they were miseducated. This phenomenon, in addition to their class position, perhaps explains why so many professionals adhere to antidialogical action. . . . Unconsciously, such persons retain the oppressor within themselves . . . they are almost unshakably convinced that it is their mission to "give" the [people] their knowledge and techniques. . . . Their programs of action (which might have been prescribed by any good theorist of oppressive action) include their own objectives, their own convictions and their own preoccupations. They do not listen to the people. (p. 153)

Freire calls upon professionals to recognize how their behavior and actions are determined from above, face the contradictions in their relationships with oppressed people, overcome their fear of their own freedom, and engage in a dialogical relationship with the oppressed. From this view, some of the discussions about empowering people can be seen for what they are: another elitist, disrespectful, paternalistic, or maternalistic means of maintaining control. Some "empowerers" do not dialogue with the people but rather proffer power from above, which, of course, can always be taken away.

An alternative view is that all people have power and through the dialogical process can begin to experience the freedom to use that power toward ending their own oppression and the oppression of others. Through this process, both leaders and people may become cooperating subjects in the historical process.

Clinical Work

Between group meetings the author had the opportunity to encounter group members on the street and arranged to go with them to secure specific services. In the course of these extragroup contacts, "clinical" issues were engaged. These ranged from the need to get treatment for alcoholism to fears they had about having AIDS, self-destructive ways in which they acted out their anger when they were denied services, and the ambivalences they had toward life and the world. They also began to share their hopefulness about their homeless group and the possibility that the group might have an effect.

In the group, members talked about writing a newsletter and other things they might try doing for themselves. This included inviting members of the Homeless Alliance, the planning organization of the Houses of Worship, and some social agencies to their group meeting. They also asked if they could participate in Homeless Alliance meetings. Homeless people had never been consulted by the Homeless Alliance. Ellen, Steve, and Sachs encouraged the group members' interest in asserting the power they had.

THE FIRST ACTION

The November monthly meeting of NHO took place after the second meeting with the homeless group. The three group leaders decided informally to raise the possibility of having an act of witness in front of the Town Hall; to open a town building now and not wait for the shelter to open. We polled NHO members informally and they agreed. We called the press. That night, in twenty-degree weather, six of us stood from 9 to 10 p.m. in front of Town Hall. We were freezing, angry, and experienced the full contradictions. We knew that five to ten homeless men and women would be out in the cold the entire night and that by 10:15 we would be warm.

Press coverage was good but town officials and the local social service agencies, including members of the Homeless Alliance, were angry. "How could you do this knowing the shelter would soon be open?" they said. We wondered why they did not do it sooner when there were questions about the shelter opening at all. Despite the Alliance members' defensiveness, some organizations and individuals cheered us on privately. They did so less often in public. NHO had not disappeared after the rent control struggle:

> The essential elements of witness which do not vary historically include: consistency between words and actions; boldness which urges the witnesses to confront existence as a permanent risk; radicalization (not sectarianism); courage to love (which far from being an accommodation to an unjust world, is rather the transformation of that world on behalf of the

increasing liberation of men [and women]); and faith in the people, since it is to them that the witness is made, although witness to the people, because of their dialectical relationship to the dominant elites, also affects the latter (who respond to the witness in their customary way).

All authentic (that is, critical) witness involves the daring to run risks, including the possibility that the leaders will not always win the immediate adherence of the people. (Freire, 1989a, p. 177)

Contradictions

There is a part of Sachs that wants to be liked. He certainly does not like to be attacked. The attack by would-be allies from the Homeless Alliance was particularly disturbing. Sachs knew NHO would have to work with them in the future. He was also very new to this small town and worried about the fallout. On the other hand, he was also making friends whom he liked and who were supportive.

The NHO leadership was creating contradictions for the professional establishment. These contradictions would increase as they sent representatives to our group and as the homeless men and women became a permanent part of the Homeless Alliance.

Practice Principles

Present talk of inadequate conditions is a cover for tolerance of repression. For the revolutionary, conditions have always appeared right. What appears in retrospect as a preliminary state or a premature situation was once for the revolutionary, a last chance to change. A revolutionary is with the desperate people for whom everything is on the line, not with those that have time. . . . Critical theory . . . rejects the kind of knowledge that one can bank on. It confronts history with the possibility which is always concretely visible within it. . . . [Humanity] is not betrayed by the untimely attempts of the revolutionaries but by the timely attempts of the realists. (Max Horkheimer, quoted in Roderick, 1986, p. 137)

Activists in small towns need to understand that it is the next-door neighbor or the folks around the corner whose interests they are opposing. In a city, anonymity is possible. Small towns do not allow for it. A local merchant angrily greeted Sachs' wife with, "Was that your husband [at the demonstration]?" The vulnerability of individual activists is another reason to work as a team. It is also a good idea to find allies who are at least marginally a part of the "establishment" or have lived in town for three or four generations. "Outsider," "New Yorker," "Jew," were easy labels to put on Sachs. Happily, they were some of the easier ones for him to wear, since he felt comfortable with and proud of the last two.

The Homeless Alliance accused the NHO leadership of making a big mistake in this action. They voiced fears that it would threaten future funding and jeopardize current programs and that NHO needed to learn that, as one member said, you could "get more with honey than vinegar." We worried whether this was true.

Clinical Work

The clinical work that was part of this action had to do with the exposure of the author's own deep-rooted fears and rational and irrational paranoia. The rent-control struggle exposed some of the individual and collective meanness that was present in the town. It scared him more than the police on horseback he met at demonstrations in New York City.

DEALING WITH IDENTIFICATION WITH THE OPPRESSOR: WORKING AT THE PSYCHOSOCIAL INTERFACE

In 1936, Anna Freud described the ego defense mechanism that she called "identification with the aggressor." In the process of development children may, as a defense against anxiety connected with fear of outside aggressors, identify with the person of the aggressor, the aggression of the aggressor, and/or the strength of the aggressor. By doing so, children avoid the anxiety connected with a vulnerable and passive position. They become active and, at least in fantasy, may see themselves as strong and in control. They may externalize their own misgivings about themselves onto someone or something in the outside world and vent their own aggression on that object (A. Freud, 1966).

In a similar manner, people who are oppressed may identify with their oppressors and attack others who, like themselves, are weak and vulnerable. It serves the oppressor well when people of oppressed classes and groups attack each other rather than joining together to fight for economic and political justice. Social welfare workers who act as intermediaries between the ruling elite and the poor contribute to this when, for example, they are involved in making decisions about the "worthy" and "unworthy" poor.

Freire (1989a) points out that leaders do well to "always mistrust the ambiguity of oppressed men, mistrust the oppressor housed in him [sic]" (p. 169). In the homeless group, it was often the case that members attacked one another, called each other "stupid," or defended the professional elite, saying such things as "You can't ask for any more" or "Come on, they [the 'unworthy homeless'] don't deserve anything. They're not even a part of our group." We also heard of the violence that took place between the group's members and other homeless people outside the group.

Parenthetically, it is worth noting that the group's only rule, one that was never violated, was no violence. The leadership never asked anyone who was drunk, angry, "inappropriate," or "uncivil" to leave. In fact, the leadership encouraged people to stay even as other group members were shouting at them "to get the hell out."

Initially, the members of NHO took a clear position against the group members' oppressor within. The way we responded to their behavior could even be viewed as an attack on the members themselves. For example, we indicated that they were acting and talking just like the workers in the agencies that had denied them services. At one point we posed the problematizing question, "What does it mean and how is it that we so often experience you as attacking one another?" The discussion that took place raised both political and psychological consciousness as they recognized how they acted out their frustrations and anger on each other and themselves rather than directing it at those who deserve it. They began to recognize that their energies could be used collectively to help one another. It was a major breakthrough that had important implications for the next phase of the group's process.

Contradictions

Were we acting as oppressors when we took a stand against the group members' oppressor within? The question suggests the answer and our reflection, which led to posing a dialogical problem, certainly led to better results. On the other hand, and this may be a rationalization, it allowed a number of group members to disagree with one another and the leadership. We all learned we could continue to work together while respectfully, though heatedly, disagreeing.

Practice Principles

Leaders must be aware of their own oppressiveness and the ambiguous relationship oppressed people have to oppression. It is only by posing this ambiguity itself as a dialogical problem that it becomes possible to develop the communion and cooperation that Freire talks about:

> In dialogical theory, at no stage can the revolutionary forgo communion with the people. Communion in turn elicits cooperation, which brings leaders and people to the fusion, described by [Che] Guevara. This fusion can exist only if revolutionary action is really human, empathic, loving, communicative, and humble, in order to be liberating. (1989a, p. 171)

It is at this level that the false dichotomy between clinical work and social action is bridged and can be seen for what it is, a way to maintain privilege and to split the profession from itself and the people with whom its progressive wing has historically worked.

THE LAST ACTION

The town's emergency shelter was scheduled to close May 1, 1990. In previous years, residents of the shelter would move to the woods, go to another town that had a year-round shelter, sleep in doorways or a dumpster, or try to move in with a sympathetic relative or friend.

In 1990, the group asked the NHO leadership to pose to the Homeless Alliance the issue of where they would go. They suggested that if a town building or other suitable dwelling was not found, they were prepared to set up tents and sleep on the town common. There was great resistance from the town's politicians and from the right wing of the social service community, which called an "emergency meeting" to berate Sachs personally after he raised the group's question and proposed action. The leadership of the Homeless Alliance neglected to invite the men and women of the homeless group to the emergency meeting, even though they said they had when they called Sachs the night before for an 8 a.m. meeting the next day. Nevertheless, money "magically" appeared for motels for any homeless person who needed it that week and the "tent in" was scaled down to a noon-to-9 p.m. vigil.

In the course of the week, the town fathers agreed to use the Town Hall as shelter from 8 p.m. to 7 a.m. until one of the local agencies could get a room in shape to house homeless people on a more permanent basis. The nine-hour vigil was successful. The group's members led the vigil. The continued threat of a tent-in, no doubt, had something to do with finding money and space to house the homeless.

Contradictions

At this stage of the group, the leadership and the group's members fused. Leadership was shared according to known abilities and interests. There was much mutual support. Sachs felt embraced when homeless men and women and his co-activists defended him at the next Homeless Alliance meeting. As one homeless man said to him, recalling Horkheimer, "Sure you make mistakes, it's because you bother doing something."

Many members of the Homeless Alliance who had resisted the action experienced contradictions. Their psychological stress was painful to watch and some of us tried to help them come to terms with it. The author suggested that it was clearly painful for them when they wanted to help and, at the same time, maintain their good relations with those in town who opposed homeless people taking control over their own lives.

Ed, a new member in the Homeless Alliance, was able to make an important contribution. He was a pacifist and an ideological ally of both NHO and the homeless group. We suggested he assume the role of the "stranger" (Simmel, 1950) and nominated him to chair the Homeless Alliance meetings at this tumultuous time.

Practice Principles

The dual principles of action and reflection are worth reiterating. The ability to share and relinquish leadership to the people is essential. Unification of the homeless with other oppressed people takes place through praxis:

> In order for the oppressed to unite, they must first cut the umbilical cord myth which binds them to the world of oppression. . . . Since the unity of the oppressed involves solidarity among them, regardless of their exact status, this unity unquestionably requires class consciousness. (Freire, 1989a, pp. 174-175)

As noted, it is also useful to have an ally who can take on a mediating position when necessary.

Clinical Work

The recognition and collective use of their power had both a therapeutic and an immunizing effect on every member of the group and other homeless and poor people who joined the vigil during its nine hours. As one usually deeply despairing and depressed man in the group said to Sachs, "I really feel good about being involved." Another often cynical woman who had not been seen in the group for some time said, "You really did it." It was good for the leaders too. Women and men do not have to identify with the aggressor or the oppressor when they affirm their own self-worth and the worth of others.

CONCLUSION AND FINAL CONTRADICTION

As of June 1990, when this was originally written, the Town Hall was open. Volunteers, including some formerly homeless men from the group, were providing security. Some of the churches mobilized to help with food, clothing, and other needs beyond what they had done in the past.

But eight new homeless people appeared. More were expected to arrive and as Ed, the pacifist, pointed out when the author was feeling overly optimistic about the gains NHO had made, "At best, it's still shit." On the other hand, no one in the group was sleeping in the woods or in a dumpster. The work that was done was a base to build on for the future.

Postscript: August 1998

Mapleton's newspaper reported that homeless men and women are being rousted from their tents and threatened with arrest for loitering throughout the town. Between 1990 and 1998, the country has moved further to the right, there has been a retrenchment of services, and poor and homeless people are increasingly under attack and are more marginalized.

Chapter 9

Introduction to Teaching

This is the seventh year (since 1992) we have taught our class together. We have also given about a dozen day-long or half-day workshops and institutes to workers, educators, and supervisors during that time. In the process of teaching the material, we have been in the process of learning. We learn from reading, from talking with students and colleagues, and from reflecting on our contradictions. In these chapters, we will describe the process in our class and the pedagogical tools and skills we have learned, developed, and find useful in our work with students. We believe they represent the best of what we have come to understand and are able to implement at this stage in our development as educators. We will also reflect back on some of the fits and starts and trials and tribulations we have encountered during the process of gaining this understanding over the past seven years.

Classroom teaching at the Smith College School for Social Work takes place over three summers. In between the summers, students do two eight-month internships at social welfare agencies around the country. In any given year, Jerry Sachs also teaches the required first- or second-year practice course and a first-year sociocultural concepts course. Fred Newdom teaches the required first-year policy courses and an elective on grant writing and lobbying. Both authors are faculty liaisons to student groups including the AIDS Coalition, the student chapter of the Bertha Capen Reynolds Society, the Jewish Students Group, and the Working Class Support Group. Both are active in a variety of antiracism groups. We are known to students, and it is typical that about 75 percent of the students who take our course have taken classes with one or both of us. We tend to get a self-selected group, but a group that has taken required courses with us, where teachers have less ability to innovate as a result of the banking system (Freire, 1989a) of education that dominates the curriculum. Nevertheless, both authors have introduced Freire into other courses through the use of codifications, readings, small group student-centered exercises, dialogue, and our, we like to think, clear values and politics. When they take our course, most students have a clear sense of us. Through their good grapevine, they have some notion of what they are going to get. Although they may not know how, they do expect that this class will be different from other courses. One way it is different, even from other courses we teach, is that we sit in the circle with students. In other courses, students sit in a circle but faculty end up behind a desk, sitting on a table or standing in front of the class. We made this decision as part of our commitment to develop a Subject to Subject relationship.

So what happens when we arrive in class the first day after their eight-month internship?

THE FIRST DAY

After welcoming the students, we ask their permission to tape the class. We explain that we use the recorded material as part of our own learning, for writing, and that we will not tape if any student, however anonymously, at any time, requests that we not do so. The students have been gracious enough to consistently grant us permission.*

We then hand out the course outline and a brief summary of who Paulo Freire was, some of Freire's central ideas, and a glossary of Freireian terms developed by Tom Heaney (1997). After that, it is time for student and faculty introductions. We ask them to say where their internships were the previous year, what moved them to sign up for our course, and what they hope to get out of the course.

---

*When we present transcriptions of the class process it will be in a slightly edited version (to maintain the flow) of what took place. However, we have not changed the order of conversation. We have sought to maintain its flavor, its spontaneity, and its energy. Occasionally, we will make theoretical and practice principle side comments. These side comments will include critical analysis of the teaching and emphasize the slow arduous process of both teaching and work with clients.

The answers are recorded on the blackboard and have been pretty standard over the years. They include: wanting to get back to the social activism they were involved in as undergrads or in other parts of their lives; to bring a larger lens to clinical work; how to go beyond Band-Dids; wanting to learn skills to advocate for clients and themselves; because the computer assigned them to the course; wanting to learn about empowerment; wanting to be clearer about how policy fits with practice; to gain more knowledge of power and empowerment; because the class fit their schedule; because a friend said they should take the class; and most flattering, if not also narcissistically gratifying, to see the "Fred and Jerry Show." We enjoy having fun as well as being serious and believe that good humor, good teaching, and good learning go together and have a central place in education.

In our own introductions, we are playful with each other, and we talk about our backgrounds in clinical work, policy, teaching, and social activism, our history in the field, and a thirty-year association that goes back to the student movement of the 1960s, settlement houses on the lower East Side of New York City in the 1970s, and now teaching our course and working with the Bertha Capen Reynolds Society.

We pick up on many of the issues and comments students raised in their introductions and current issues such as welfare reform, licensure, and homelessness that we are actively involved in for pay and/or as volunteers. For example, it is typical for students to raise issues related to managed care driving their practice as clinicians. This quickly gives us the opportunity to underline the role of economics in the creation of contradictions in agency policy and clinical practice.

After the introductions, we recognize the contradictions in the class itself. In a college or university setting, faculty have more power than students. If we want to make it sound nicer, we can say that faculty and students have different roles, for example, we grade them, we design the curriculum and the course outline in advance and without their consultation, and so on. We then ask rhetorically, "Who controls the course and who controls the dialogue?" We introduce Freire's ideas about the difference between Subject-to-Subject and Subject-to-Object dialogue. We recognize that there is a contradiction for all of us upon entering the room—that the class setting and structure is in contradiction to the values we hold. We also suggest some of the ways we try to level the playing field.

This past year, we introduced Ira Shor's (1996) experiment with his after-class group (ACG). We invited students, on a voluntary basis, to meet with us for lunch after each of our classes. We meet to debrief the class and examine and reflect on ideas and problems. We bring ideas that they generate and/or changes they want to suggest back to the class for discussion. Our hope is that the ACG provides a forum for students to have more give and take with us as equals. Nine students (out of an enrollment of twenty-one) attended after the first class and between eight and ten students after that. We agreed that, at the beginning of each class, after we asked for questions and comments, someone who attended the ACG would report on the meeting. This was done so that everyone could discuss the issues, topics, and concerns that were raised. After the fourth ACG, students who had attended the group requested that they meet alone every other time. Their assertion of power and their recognition that they too often deferred to the instructors, even in the ACG, was most welcome.

After this opening, we ask students to reflect on their experiences at Smith before our class. We recognize with them the school's attempt to socialize them into Smith's conception of a professional. The "Smith way" is similar to the approach of other schools. The dichotomy between clinical work and social action is rarely bridged. We discuss the norms, values, and beliefs that the school has imparted. Indeed, as one student put it, their education until now has actively tried to maintain the dichotomy so that social activism would not "contaminate" their clinical work. We recognize out loud that they may feel that what they have been taught may not be fully internalized in a way that feels comfortable. We acknowledge that here we are telling them there is yet another way. This class is, at least in part, in contradiction to what they have paid for and, with many, gone into debt to learn. We acknowledge that what we teach may be seen by some of them as refreshing though problematic. Other students may experience the class content as an assault on their professional selves (Mead, 1934). These are selves that they have, often with difficulty, if not painfully, been in the process of developing.

We also let them know that we do not want to throw the baby out with the bathwater. We suggest that much of what they have learned is valuable and merely needs to be tweaked and broadened, not thrown out. We share with them that we have a distinct set of values. When these values are operationalized in practice, they may also contradict a good deal of what they have learned. For example, we quickly explode the belief that a theory can be value free or that theories can be implemented objectively and neutrally without paying attention to their values. As always, we leave time for comments, cross talk, and questions.

With this relatively didactic base, we introduce the concept of problematizing phenomena, how problematizing can be a means to facilitate meaningful dialogue and create critical consciousness. For example, in working with a mother on welfare, rather than trying to problem solve, they might begin a dialogue with her. It is important to understand what it means for her to be on welfare. In the dialogue, we would question how it shapes her in the context of her world at this moment in time. We observe with them that this pointing to the thing itself, with the welfare mother, is phenomenological. This problematizing is intended to develop dialogue, deep reflection, and a critical attitude with the recipient about her place in the social world. This new view of her taken-for-granted world might then lead to personal and collective action with other recipients, advocates, and the worker.

To further engage students as Subjects in a problematizing process, we ask them to pick something from the list on the board that they presented in their introductions so that we can together look deeply into the meanings of what they identified. This past year, the students picked "becoming a well-rounded social worker" from the list on the board. We asked the class what that meant to them.

A student said that it means "not getting stuck in one way of doing things." It was suggested that this was a negative way of putting it. We asked her if she could turn it around. She picked up on this and said "having many ways of doing things as a social worker." We then asked for examples, suggesting that the question was not just for her. Another student offered that it meant "using different perspectives, psychodynamic theory, keeping in mind an ecological perspective, person-in-environment, as well as keeping in mind roles and different kinds of tools. . . ." We pointed out that this was "OK, but very abstract," and asked, "What kinds of tools?" Yet another student, "avoiding" our question, spoke of "understanding policy, understanding clinical work and how they all affect each other." Again, one of us said, "OK, but still abstract," and added that "if two more people are abstract, we will need to ask how come we need to be so abstract."

At this point, students were able to be somewhat less abstract and talked about such things as mobilizing opposition to welfare reform time limits, and having experiences in a range of practice settings and with a range of clients.

Eventually, we picked up on the abstractness of the responses and asked in a problematizing way, "What did they make of the fact that they were being so abstract and that more often than not, in the curriculum, things were kept fairly abstract rather than concrete?" A student responded to this and suggested that "if you're concrete, you're more accountable." We asked the students to say more about that.

A student suggested that it was "the students' lack of experience." We replied that the "faculty do it [we're abstract] too" (laughter in class).

Another student said, "To make it all concrete, it would take a lot more time and effort. It would be great if we could do that, but academia doesn't do that."

F: Says who?*
S: In classes.
J: Maybe in other places but we'd like to support being concrete [laughter in class] and I think you were getting to something when you said, "You're accountable!"
S: I agree, yeah, you might be wrong or, if things don't work out, somehow it's going to fall apart. What then?

Another student suggested that being concrete might mean that you would fail. We wondered aloud, "So what if you fail?"

---

* Throughout, Fred Newdom will be represented by "F"; Jerry Sachs by "J"; and students by "S," unless we specify a fictional name.

Yet another student made the observation that "clinical social work is a very theory-based practice, that we're taught to think in the abstract."

A student added, "And we want to!"

At this point, Sachs shared the concreteness he tries to get across to his practice class when he suggests to them that "clients come to us, say something, and then it's our turn. Our turn may be silence, or to ask a question, or to be abstract, but whatever we say, however we respond, it is in concrete words. . . . In this class, we like to problematize what is said and, in that spirit, what you said, 'more accountable' and 'might fail if concrete,' what do those things mean?"

S1: Being concrete, how hard it is to do. If you go against the grain in the abstract, if you go against the grain in your real life, you may be really hitting a wall.

S2: Yeah, if you say something concrete, it's something they can nail you on. That's exposure. You're vulnerable out there. What are you going to do? So when you're vague and abstract, it's yada yada yada.

J: [with a bit of sarcasm, trying to emphasize the clinical nature of what they've been saying] Are you saying this is a psychological defense? [laughter in class]

S3: Yeah, a lot of it is fear.

J: Yes, not only other people can nail you, but, if you're sensitive, and get down to it yourself, it can produce what Paulo Freire calls an "act of self-violence." Because you begin to see that if this is what I thought I was doing, in this nice abstract way, and that's safe, but this is what I am really doing, concretely, which doesn't quite fit with that, I'm in a contradiction. That's painful. Who needs it? Better the old defenses. Y'know, a little collusion between faculty and students, between supervisors and students, sometimes even between clients and workers. It's safe. No one has to be accountable.

F: It is easier to talk in the abstract about social justice than talk about going out on the street and doing something about it. With the client, on the ground, face to face, one on one, in the real world. Abstract talk loses something and really is a good defense.

After the class break, we go over the course syllabus and the required paper. Next, we discuss our membership in a value-based profession and elaborate on the values we presented in Chapter 2. Then, we begin to tie in our theory base to our values. Theory and values must be congruent and both must be congruent with practice. Our question to them and to ourselves is, "When a worker or teacher says or does something, is what they say or do in sync with or in contradiction to their theory and/or their values?"

If there is a contradiction, it is necessary to consider the meanings and motives involved. What should be done next if one hopes to be faithful to one's values and theory? We point out the usefulness of two people teaching this course. One helps the other recognize contradictions that may be too painful to see alone. When contradictions are painful, they may be repressed because of false consciousness or anxiety or countertransference. The first class ended here.

Chapter 10

A Case Discussion

The second class began by discussing the wish to keep things concrete rather than abstract. The class agreed that they would try to be concrete, and we asked that they hold us to the same standard.

We then picked up on something, Lori, a student, had raised in the previous class. She asked, "What if you choose to be in conflict? Is that a contradiction?" and gave the example of her work with a "man who had a tremendous amount of guilt about having sexual encounters with males in the past. It was really hard for me not to say something like, 'That's OK, I don't have a problem.' My value was that same-sex sex is fine. But he felt guilty, so we had a session where I let my values come out and it turned out that that was not helpful to him. So the rest of the time, I chose to be in conflict and I didn't pretend that I was someone who believed otherwise. I wonder, in retrospect, if it would have been better never to reveal my values, that same-sex sex is OK, and great, fabulous sometimes, because that was counterproductive for him. So that was what I said."

We problematized Lori's issue for the class by asking, "What does it mean for our student, for the guy, for the society, and are there more than the two possibilities that Lori suggested, i.e., sharing or not sharing one's values? What do you all think?"

A student responded, asking about the worker role. "Is it being a neutral party, recognizing that our values, history, etc. were going to influence the work either overtly or covertly?" Yet another student asked for more information about the case. Though reasonable, it is also possible that these "abstract" questions were a way to avoid what we tried to problematize.

Lori then suggested it was complicated but that her intervention caused a rift, because it challenged her "client's values and the values of his family who he was close to. At that point it was unfathomable to him. For me to say that was like I was an alien. Instead of me following his process, it really made a huge rift. And interesting because he's a very strong person and intelligent. He recognized that some people, meaning him, don't agree with him but 'for me' [for him] this is a sin. So he was able to reframe it but it took a week and he missed a session."

Another student empathized, saying that if she had a disagreement with a client, she would feel, "Oh no, I'm going to lose a client."

We pointed out that we do not own the client and that the client is not ours to lose. We also recognized, in a clinical way, that the student's anticipation of losing the client may have been related to anxiety about loss of object-love or superego anxiety related to the fact that she (the student) may have done something wrong.

Lori: I felt that it's not bad that he saw my values. That was valuable, but what I question is how I let it come out. There's no way I can go back and see how it would have gone. But I wonder. . . .

S: As therapists, we want to make a client feel better, seeing someone so upset and knowing they don't have to live that way. We know another reality. But that's invalidating to that person's reality.

Lori: Exactly. That's exactly how I felt. I had this impulse, because he was in such tremendous pain, for me to say, "Wait a minute."

F: We need to tease out what's the contradiction in this. Because, from your description of it today, I wonder what you saw the contradiction as being.

Lori: After this rift, at times, I did bite my tongue. There were times when I tried to monitor that impulse. And that felt like a conflict to me.

J: What I hear is two values going on simultaneously. One is your value to be open about this issue and that you have your own values, that same-sex sex is fine. And the second value relates to a value that you have about the therapeutic process, which says you should stay with the client and be empathic and go where they are. And you felt the first one created a contradiction with the second. I would suggest that happens to us all the time because we have multiple values, some of which conflict with one another. The question I would raise is, when you saw that happen with him, it was your turn. He had a very strong reaction, one that you wished he might not have had but one that he, in fact, had. I want to go back to a key Freirian word, "dialogue." When you see that reaction in him, can you continue the dialogue at that moment? Clearly it took a week to get back to it, and he fortunately was able to get back to it, but I would suggest that, even at that moment, one could get into his reaction. A worker could say, "You have a reaction to what I just said, a pretty strong reaction. Say more. Let's verbalize it right here and now. I'm open to it." He can talk about his value, thinking this is sinful. And one can even go into that in greater depth. "What makes it sinful for you? Where did you learn that? What's the history of it for you? What did you imagine about what I said? Where do you think that's coming from?" We can follow his fantasy about us, so that this can be opened up in a clinical therapeutic kind of way. That might lead, at some point, to social action. Because he did say, even a week later, "I do know that some people out there have a different view than I do." He at least knows there is another world outside himself. It might lead to some connection for him with that world. Maybe not. That's his choice. But maybe.

Lori: We did talk about that and, at one point, I asked if he wanted to see a priest. That's totally against my values. But he didn't want that. He came to a middle ground. I think I see what you're saying.

S: So, in asserting ourselves with clients we are giving them an opportunity to try out our reality. In that way, it expands their minds to think of things in a different way, in dialogue.

J: Well, I'm not sure I'd put it that way. Though I wouldn't be antagonistic to the way you're putting it. I think what I would say is, along with Freire, that we are going back to what has been suggested. That we are who we are. There is no possibility to do otherwise. If we bury it, unconsciously, it's going to come out some other way, anyway. And it is more honest, with the person we're working with, to say, at an appropriate moment, what we believe and our values, so long as we are not demanding that they share those values. As long as we are willing to be in dialogue with them about our values, as well as their values, and how they, in this therapeutic situation, touch one another. Perhaps we create some conflict. The message we want to send to them, at the end of the day, is that no matter what we say to each other, we can talk about it more. We have the next time we meet or later this time and it continues to be opened up. We want to keep the system open to dialogue and, so far as possible, never close it down on our side and help them keep it open on their side.

At this point, we discussed the timing of when to share our values. This is tricky given the power difference between a worker and a client. It is useful to explore the reason a client wants to know our values at a particular point in the therapeutic process. What is the meaning of the client's question about our values? For example, a client may be using the question as a resistance to looking at something else more deeply or may be just interested in knowing where a worker is at or, in an overdetermined way, have both and other motives simultaneously. We emphasized the need to inquire into the meanings of the question. "That's a first step before sharing what our values are." To do less would potentially foreclose our, and more important, the client's, understanding of the question. Lori then questioned what we said.

Lori: You're just moving the time [when you state your values]. The conflict is still there!

J: I would not be biting my tongue. I would be doing what I think would be valuable therapeutic work with the person to find out the meaning of the question. Then, if they understand, sometimes the question will drop away. Because what's important is how come they asked. And sometimes, it won't drop away. In which case, I would hope to give them a forthright and clear answer. Then I would follow up with what they think of my answer because that has meaning too. The dialogue is kept open.

F: The tension is between biting my tongue and not being assertive, saying what I believe and honoring the client's right to control the therapeutic process. If that's the tension, one is more about "I feel a need to speak up" and the other is "I feel a need to work where the client is." If it were to be posed that way, as a question, I think most people would say, "I feel a need to work where the client is." Because, at some point, dialogue may bring you to a place where your values are something the client really wants to have in the mix.

Lori: It's an issue of a calculated risk to disclose. If I did it earlier in the treatment he would have left, bolted. But, in my impulse to make it better, that's where I think I didn't do the best and wish I could see it more as a calculated risk and let it out slowly. It was lucky that he didn't bolt.

J: I would say that's true but also that you may have known internally, on some unconscious level, that he wouldn't bolt.

The student recognized her need to "make it better" rather than explore the client's feelings of sinfulness. In hindsight, the instructor observed that he may have wanted to make the student feel better rather than fully explore her motivation. It is anxiety provoking to sit with someone else's anxiety. The conflicts that create another's anxiety tap into our own anxiety. Workers and teachers also have needs to "make it better."

Lori: Yeah, you're right.

J: The question is the exploration of his feelings about "sinful." If we jump ahead about three months' worth of sessions, it may be that, in his own dialogue, as part of the therapeutic process, he may begin to see, in a clearer way, where this value of his came from. It is in contradiction to his behavior, and he may come to ease up on himself. The guilt may ease up and he may even say, "My parents or some other people in my environment were oppressive to me, not only in that way, but in a whole slew of ways." At which point, one can ask the question, "Is there anything you'd like to do about this?" This moves you to a social action position. Again, the timing of that is important. I would not come in first thing and say, "What do you want to do about this?" This would take us off to the races.

S: How is this problematizing?

J: Two levels: problematizing in class by asking it as a question. So we discovered two sets of values going on here. We have more information about the situation, which gives us a better understanding of it. This may then lead us to do different kinds of actions with the client. If we were to do a role play, we might ask, "How else might we approach this with the client that would not do violence to our own values? Is there another way to go?" And we're just taking a look to see if that's possible and want to say out loud, "Sometimes it may not be." We make choices and dialogue about the choices.

Here we recognize the slow, arduous process of both teaching and work with clients and the necessity to constantly feed back information and experiences for dialogue.

J: This is consciousness raising. His family, his friends imposed values upon him about this issue. He may discover that in terms of psychological consciousness raising. And he may also find that they didn't discover this all by themselves. This came from the larger society which imposed it upon them which imposed it upon him. We know that this is an awareness that can come out of problematizing what he's bringing to the therapeutic process.

Here the instructor would have done well to talk to socialization rather than imposition. It would have been more neutral and less pejoratively value laden.

Lori: That's exactly what we did [but] didn't get to the social action part.
J: But, if you had that in your consciousness, at some appropriate time, you could have connected him to a gay rights group. Could he have taken you up on that?

The question might be raised here whether the instructor was pushing overly hard for the social action component at this point, which the student again, in her way, questioned.

Lori: It would have to be a long time.
J: We're patient, I hope.

In this comment, the teacher backs off and agrees that "social action, like good therapeutic work, may take a long time, a year, five years, fifteen years. Fred and I have been at it thirty-five years and we're still not at our goals. So, this is a long process and you do it incrementally, by successive approximations, and we do the best we can." At this point, another student got very concrete in a way that led to a role play.

S: I still have a question. When a client does ask you the question, what do you say?

J: I might say to you, "What brings you to ask me that question at this point in our work?"

S: Well, we've been talking about it and I was just wondering what you thought.

J: OK, and what do you imagine?

S: About what?

J: About what I might answer.

S: I don't know. That's why I ask.

J: It is true that you don't know and, at some point after the discussion, we should talk about that and I would likely [teacher hedging his bets] share with you what I think. But, what is important now is what's your best guess? What's your fantasy?

S: I guess I could go two ways.

J: Well, go one of the ways. [in an aside to the class] Which doesn't mean the client isn't ambivalent and might, in fact, go both ways in their head.

S: I don't know. So that's why I asked.

J: So what are the possibilities of what you might hear from me?

S: That you think it's worse.

J: Uhhuh, and what if I thought it was worse?

S: [in an aside to the whole class] Anyone want to take my place? [laughter in class] You would hate me, think it's gross and think I was a horrible person.

J: And if I were to hate you and think it's gross and that you were a horrible person, that would be a terrible thing for a worker who was working with you to do. If I thought that.

Here the instructor, in an effort to move things along, intervened in a stronger way than he would in actual work. Usually, he works more slowly.

S: Well, I feel that this relationship is so important to me. I couldn't handle that.

J: But, if I thought that, what would you do and why should you handle it?

S: I would be crushed.

J: How come you would be crushed if you thought I had a problem with it?

S: Because you're the only person who knows.

J: Who knows?

S: These feelings I have.

J: But what would you think of a person who you've shared this with, this intimate thing, about yourself, [who] thought that this was really gross, what would you think of such a person?

S: Why can't you just answer the question? [laughter in class]

J: That's a good question and I will but [laughter in class] what would you think of such a person who, when you're sharing some of your most intimate feelings, would think that those feelings are gross?

S: You talked about other things and were right about them. Then you'd be right about me. Think I'm really gross.

In the role play, we can note the client's projection and the transferential implications of what he said, that is: Who in the client's past thought this or other things were gross?

J: You think that would be OK? What do you think about the continuation of this relationship, if I thought that?

S: Hard.

J: Hard? How come it would be hard?

S: Constantly rejecting.

J: Why would you want to be with someone who was constantly rejecting?

S: That's the best I can do.

J: That's the best you can do? Boy, that would be unfortunate if that were true. [Here the worker holds out hope and poses a dialectic, but one might also ask whether he is again just "making it better," depriving the client of the opportunity to fully experience the pain connected with rejection and opening past rejections.]

S: I think it is.

At this point, the instructor playfully attempted to begin concluding the role play with the following comment.

J: So that sounds like what you talked about three weeks ago, with staying in the other relationship which is just like this. [laughter in class] And we're off to hopefully decent kinds of therapeutic work. I am also implying here that this is one of the dumbest things a therapist could do. And the person should get out of the relationship if I had such thoughts. And I would say that to my best friend. No one should be in that kind of crazy therapeutic relationship with someone who thinks what they are experiencing is gross when you're not hurting anyone else. So, I am sending, without being explicit, a message about what my values are.

S: What if someone is doing something gross?

J: If someone is beating on a kid, for example, turn them in to DSS. That's the law. They should know that up front. If work continues with that person, you need to get at the meaning of their hitting a child and that there are severe consequences to that. They need to know that one of those consequences is that I'll turn them in.

S: Does it send the message that you're disapproving?

F: Yes, but it doesn't send the message that "you're one of the lowest life forms existing on the planet and I can't stand being in the same room as you." So it talks to disapproving of the behavior but wanting to work with the person.

S: You could always fall back on your role as a mandated reporter.

J: But saying "I'll turn you in" is taking responsibility. It's between me and him, not some abstract mandated reporter, the court. It's me. I'm going to turn you in. Face to Face [Subject to Subject because my values require that].

S: But there is the tendency to put the responsibility on the court.

J: That's true, but that's not the most useful way of working and we could problematize that if we wanted to.

Lori then came back to the question she raised in the previous class and why we grabbed onto it. "I'm wondering what it was that gave you guys that glimmer, when I asked you last time what you were hoping, what dialogue were you hoping to get to, based on contradictions?"

This gave us an opportunity to again talk to how we attempt to play out our values, theory, and practice in the class.

J: What gave us the glimmer was that there was a contradiction and we never know in advance where we are going to go.

F: But we did know that our stance is that everything is something from which we can teach and learn. And if the issue is contradiction and we're working on contradiction. Let's go with where Lori is and see where that goes. It could have been a ten-minute conversation. [It actually turned out to be a forty-five-minute conversation.]

L: I was wondering whether there was a particular thing you were hunting for?

Here, we note the student's previous classroom socialization and, in that light, reasonable expectations.

J: Let's introduce another notion here, because if we had known in advance exactly where we wanted to go with this, it would be what Freire calls a "banking model." We open your head and pour in the knowledge. [laughter in class] But we'd like to think that the discussion that we're having here, which is not preprogrammed, is a better way of doing it. [Another student then moved to another tangent.]

S: Another issue is when you thought you weren't in conflict, and it comes to your attention that you were. We place a lot of value on knowing what we're doing.

J: Hopefully you think about it yourself, with a friend, a good supervisor who can problematize it with you. Some of it may be rooted in countertransference. Some may be rooted in your political history. But that's to be discovered. And there is action and reflection and action and reflection and action and reflection and this is the reflection part which will move you to the next action which may be different than when you were in conflict. Folks [meaning clients] out there are very forgiving when we make mistakes.

Another student introduced the idea of differences between conflict and contradiction. That question gave us an opportunity to clarify that contradiction is a conflict that centers on our values, in relation to theory and practice. We again noted that values themselves may be in conflict. When they are, contradictions are inevitable. Dialogue about that tension with oneself and with the client is useful. In addition, we underline our premise that there are clinical dimensions to social action and social action dimensions to clinical work. At the appropriate place and time, they both need to be engaged.

For example, with the client we were talking about, he might eventually say that he would like to go to a gay rights group but that he is afraid they will not like him there "because I come from this religious background." Now that piece of social action also has a clinical dimension. His concerns about being liked and the move toward political action may open up the clinical issue just as a clinical issue can open a political issue, and we want to be open to both.

We also emphasize how much our work is with ourselves, examining our work in relation to our values. We have to look at ourselves in relation to gender, class, and race issues. If we take our values seriously, this is a necessity. That is a difficult and never-ending process.

Chapter 11

Codifications

A codification is a representation of the learner's day-to-day situations. It can be a photograph, a drawing or even a word. As a representation, the photograph or word is an abstraction that permits dialogue leading to an analysis of the concrete reality represented. Codifications mediate between reality and its theoretical context, as well as between educators, and learners who together seek to unveil the meanings of their existence. (Heaney, 1997, p. 8)

The coding of an existential situation is the representation of that situation showing some of its constituent elements in interaction. Decoding is the critical analysis of the coded situation. (Freire, 1989a, p. 96)

INTRODUCTION TO CODIFICATIONS

As an educator, Freire (1989a) used codes as a tool to engage the most meaningful generative themes in the life of a group with whom he was working. He used the term "'generative' because (however [themes] are comprehended and whatever action they may evoke) they contain the possibility of unfolding [other] themes, that, in their turn, call for new tasks to be fulfilled" (p. 92). Many codes Freire used were in the form of drawings. This was the starting place to teach reading to groups of illiterate people with whom he worked in communities in Brazil. Codifications are the starting point for dialogue between members of a community group and between members of a group and the educators/facilitators. The aim of dialogue is to illuminate "ideas, values, concepts, and hopes, as well as the obstacles" (p. 91) members of a group face in their everyday existence. It is a starting place to illuminate the world.

In class, we begin by handing out a codification developed by the Canadian social worker Bonnie Burstow (1991) and her class. It is a "Codification on Native Americans Subjected to White People's Schooling" (see Figure 11.1).

We explain that a codification could be a drawing similar to the one in front of them, but could also be a song, a poem, a dance, or some other representation of a community. What is important is that the themes represented in a codification are tied to the daily experience of the individuals in the community being engaged. However, the dialogue that grows out of the process of decoding can move beyond local community concerns to national or even international concerns. These national and international issues can then be connected back to local concerns. Codifications are another way to begin to problematize situations. The critical analysis of a code can lead to conscientization.

The use of codifications with illiterates is contrasted with their use with superliterates who teach or study at universities. With illiterate people, codes are used to teach reading and develop "abstract" dialogue about concrete situations in the world of a cultural community. With superliterates, codes can be used to get people out of their heads and, paradoxically, help them, through an abstract picture, to become more concrete and enter into dialogue.

After this introduction, students are asked what they see. What does the picture of the Native American class reveal?

This past year a student began, "What jumps out is the important dates." Another student observed, "Very threatening, the principal over there, and the teacher is holding a big stick." Other students asked about the Canadian flag, the birds outside the class, and the clock on the wall.

We then asked, "What do these things mean? For whom are the dates important?" Students quickly responded, noting that "the dates represent invasion [indeed a cultural invasion] more than discovery." "The clock represents measurement, punctuality, and forced structured time." Yet another student contrasted the "controls in the class" to the "birds' freedom outside the class."

FIGURE 11.1. Codification on Native Americans Subjected to White People's Schooling

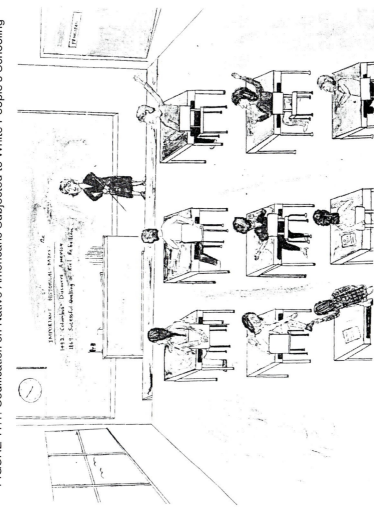

Source: Burstow, B. (1991). Freirian codifications and social work education, *Journal of Social Work Education, 27*(2), 196-207. Copyright ©1991 Council on Social Work Education, Alexandria, VA.

They had quickly been able to identify several major themes and issues that Native American students or their parents might also pick up on if they had been presented with this drawing. An educator/worker/facilitator could encourage dialogue about these themes. The dialogue could lead to an individual's or group's feelings about the world, to a deeper understanding of the world, and possibly to social action to change the world. For example, a worker could engage the theme of the students being treated as Objects and that they are named and contained by a dominating culture. Group members would be encouraged to express their feelings about these phenomena, to act as Subjects, to name themselves and assert their freedom.

A student in class then noticed another detail. "The IQ test is a political issue that might come out of this. Students are ranked, and the creation of IQ tests, the proliferation of IQ tests, is something that has a great deal of political significance." Another student added, "The IQ test itself is based not on who they are, or where they are, but on the historical dates on the blackboard. That's probably part of the IQ test." The political action would be to find new ways to engage these students and create culturally syntonic ways to teach, "test," and "evaluate" them.

Pessimistically, another student added, "What really bothers me about the picture is that all the kids are totally swallowing what's up there. No one is getting upset, or saying, 'Who are you to say that these are important dates?' or anything else, like discovering America. What about the people who were already there? They're just totally OK."

In response, an instructor noted that there are a "couple of kids on the left side who are resisting the program." That "it is not unusual for oppressed people in the face of the oppressor to put on an inauthentic smile to please the oppressor, protect themselves, and subvert the oppressor." In addition, codifications are not meant to be set in stone. A group of Native students could be asked what they think the messages are in the notes that the kids are passing to one another. Fred wondered, "Are these kids who just can't sit still, or does the note say, 'Meet me outside, after this piece of oppression ends, and we'll plan the revolution'" (laughter in class). With native students, we might ask: "What does the note say?" Groups are encouraged to change a codification or develop one of their own. For example, Native students or their parents might be asked to write the messages they would want to send to each other in the notes.

SOME ADDITIONAL IDEAS ABOUT CODES AND THEIR USES

Facilitators should always come with lots of blank paper and lots of magic markers. To help a group move into dialogue about a codification, Freire (1989b) and Burstow (1991) suggest a number of questions. These include:

- What's happening here?
- Does anything about the picture bother you?
- What are the contradictions in the picture?
- Who has the power?
- Who wins?
- Who loses?
- Who is helping?
- Who is sabotaging?
- In whose interest is this happening?
- Are there other people who need to be in this picture who are not shown?
- How can the situation be changed?

Codifications are tools that can open up dialogue, reflection, and action among groups of people, and between the workers and the people with whom they work. Codifications can be used clinically with individuals, groups, or families. For example, a family that had difficulty talking could be encouraged to draw parts of their life and their environment. The family would dialogue about their drawings and/or about the process of developing the picture they drew. They could draw pictures of their past, their present, and what they imagined and/or hoped their future would be. Individual drawings and those which were collectively developed would then be compared.

Codifications are worked with in a single meeting or over time. Intrapersonal, interpersonal, and political themes and issues exist within the codes people draw. All issues and themes are addressed and engaged. For example, each of the Native students in the codification has a psychology and so does the teacher. The interpersonal relations between students and between the students and the teacher could be addressed. Finally, and simultaneously, political issues and social action issues are addressed. What is essential is that the leader be flexible and the choices individuals, groups, and families make come out of dialogue. The choice of what to draw is not imposed from above. That would contradict our values as well as go against the clinical rule of starting where the client is.

Near the end of the introduction to codifications in 1998, a student asked, "If we were to do codifications of Smith School for Social Work, would it be things we see as part and parcel of the school, or things that need changing?" Simultaneously the teachers said, "YES!" The class laughed at our response. The question was the perfect segue to the exercise that we hoped they would do in the next class.

CODIFICATIONS OF STUDENTS' EXPERIENCES IN SUMMER CLASSES AND IN THE FIELD

The remainder of this chapter focuses on four codifications that were created by students in the summer of 1998. The reflections and dialogue about these codes took place over two classes, but content in the codes, and particularly the idea of "dangerous thoughts," was brought up in all later classes. The following is an abridged and edited version of what took place. We believe it captures the main themes and issues that were raised as well the spirit and energy in the class.

We start by asking the class to count off into four groups. The codification exercise (Exercise 1 below) is handed out. Two of the groups are asked to draw number 1 and the other two groups to draw number 2. Sheets of flip chart paper and a large selection of magic markers are provided. The groups are asked to select a presenter for when they come back from their work and all group members and the class as a whole are encouraged to make comments. The groups then go off to work for about twenty-five to thirty minutes.

* * *

Exercise 1

1. Develop a codification of your experiences at the School related to clinical work and social action during the past summers. Highlight how these two facets of social work were integrated and/or the contradictions that you experienced.
2. Develop a codification of your experiences in the field related to clinical work and social action. Highlight how these two facets of social work were integrated and/or the contradictions that you experienced.

* * *

When the groups return, their codifications are hung on the wall and they are asked, "Who wants to begin?" This year Sarah, the presenter from group 1, began (see Figure 11.2). "It's the Smith Experience. The first one is our first summer [laughter in class]. Inside of that tornado, I don't know if you can see there's the college, there's books, there's homes, there's people, dogs, and cats. And then by the second summer we're kinda feeling like Gumby. We're stretched and pulled in all directions. And Gumby's eyes are clocks. Because time is of the essence. Like Dali's clock melting. And then, by the third summer, of course, we are all these wonderful octopuses who have enough tentacles to do it all. Of course the clocks are still looming all over us, those jellyfish clocks."

At this point, other students noticed the eyes, the dollar signs, and the intense, almost grimacing smiles. They commented on the expressiveness of the drawing and the role of money in their lives as they are about to graduate. Comments were offered on how stretched they were. The class questioned whether the optimism of the last part of the drawing, the octopus who could handle so many tasks, was real or whether, at this stage of the summer, with a thesis to be finished, some of them were really very stressed.

Sarah noted that "the smile was intended to be drawn, not stressed. It's supposed to be a loose smile." To which another member of her group said, "But it was impossible to draw." Jerry then

FIGURE 11.2. The Smith Experience

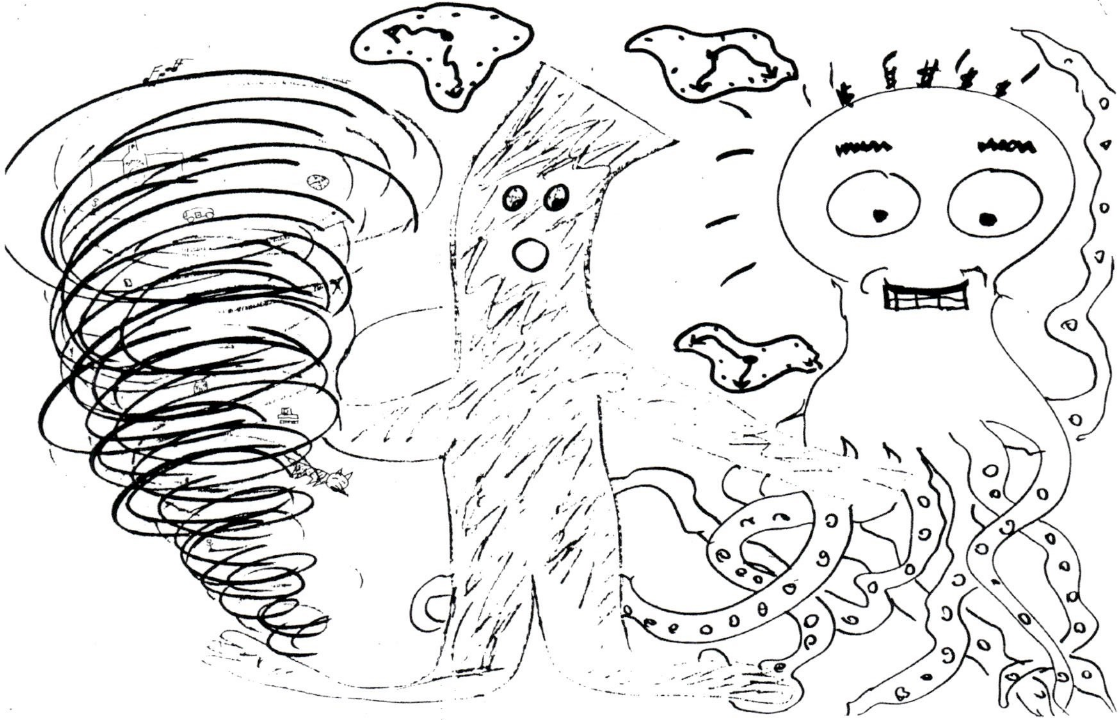

made a clinical point observing that "the unconscious never lies" (laughter in class). Other students then added that the eyes look wide open, as though they were taped open, stunned, as in the film *A Clockwork Orange*.

The instructors then commented on how the codification might be used. "What we would want to do is pick up one of your comments that seemed full of feeling and meaning. For example, there are different characterizations of the eyes, from a 'deer in headlights being stunned' to 'the eyes are wide open.' These different characterizations are open to multiple interpretations. There are lots of ways to think about the eyes and there were a number of different ways people saw the eyes. There was a lot of feeling behind what people saw even though the people who drew the code may not have intended it." After a short silence, Sarah and other students responded.

Sarah: It was also about what we left out. We had a discussion about putting in words at the bottom that would literally talk about all the things we felt. That we were being stretched, but we felt that was too literal, and that everybody would understand and see their common experience. So that just explains the experience that the eyes would be bugging out.

S1: To me they look like they are afraid and kind of anxious.

S2: The unconscious piece. My eyes have finally been open to something, whether it's a negative reality or positive reality. You're finally seeing stuff. The tornado doesn't have any eyes. Gumby, the eyes are open but smaller, and all of a sudden there's all of this awareness around you.

S3: The Gumby looks like, "Oh I'm not sure about this." It looks like I finally do see it. And the eyes can also be internal eyes too. Because the first summer, for some the second summer, seeing things, trying to figure things out for yourself, and the third summer, there's a lot of things I need to learn.

S4: Yeah, yeah. It's the real world.

S1: It's not just the real world.

S5: I wonder, can it also be getting beyond yourself? In a way even though the eyes are very prominent, the lines of the marker are much more finely done. So the actual shape of the body doesn't come out as much. So it could be like getting out of yourself, or outside of your perspective, or whatever.

J: [attempting to move things, perhaps prematurely, along] There were these dollar signs, someone mentioned, hanging over the octopus's head.

S6: Or our head.

S7: Loans and debt.

S8: Like the first figure is completely out of control. The middle is kind of like, uhhh, and the end is like trying to be in control, but not being able to do it. Like trying to grasp more than eight different things at once.

Later the class was asked if they could "identify the clinical and social action issues that were present in the drawing."

S: Yes! [laughter in class]

S7: Well, it makes me think of the money as a huge force on the octopus. Y'know, because it has to go and figure out how to pay back the loans and it's a driving force.

Here the instructors brought in some history related to social work education that the students knew almost nothing about. The 1960s and early 1970s were described. The class learned that most students in training had scholarships, full tuition, often a stipend, and that some public agencies paid full salaries to their workers as they studied for their MSWs. The students were incredulous at the difference between that experience and their own.

Here again, we engaged the students' lack of historical knowledge. Both personal and political issues were opened. This revealed the historical world of social work education for students and showed that their taken-for-granted world (Schutz, 1967) of social work education was not always "taken for granted." This decoding illustrated how a codification could create meaningful dialogue with a client or community groups that bridged the dichotomy between individual intrapsychic work and work that had implications for acting on the social institutional world.

The class took its break here with the sense that we would move on to the second codification, one that focused on their field experiences (see Figure 11.3).

FIGURE 11.3. Interactions in the Field

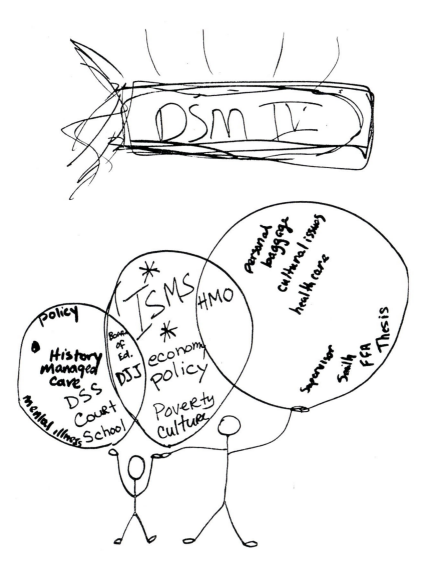

Ann [the student presenter from group 2]: It's the one we call interactive because we started to fill in the circles above the people. We left it open for people to add to those circles. And I think we're saying that the people in the bottom are the client and the social worker. The small one is the client. The other one is the social worker. And I think we did it that way in terms of how we feel. Our interpretation of how we feel. Like the social workers feel small, within the agency, especially as an intern. You feel on the bottom of the ladder. And yes, we feel that the clients feel even smaller than we do. So that's our representation of how small we feel, and how the client sees himself. And the balls are kind of the pressures we feel and they're laying on us and the differences are that the person to the left is the client and the things that the clients themselves will deal with. The one in the middle is what we both deal with as a client and as a social worker in terms of society, societal pressures, and on top is the DSM (*Diagnostic and Statistical Manual*).

Joe [another student in group 2]: The first circle is what we felt the client deals with, managed care, DSS, court system, schools, policies. That's the first one, what the client's holding. The second is what the client and the social worker are holding up together and that's more the societal issues, economic policy, poverty, culture, the "isms." The third one is what the intern is holding up for themselves which is the school, the supervisor, the FFAs (Faculty Field Advisors), health care, the other issues. We kind of left it that people could come and fill in because there's other issues. In terms of the circle in the middle you could put in violence, crime. . . . There's other things we could put in. But it's just to start a dialogue about what goes on.

Liz [a third student in group 2]: We would have liked to draw other things but we didn't have time.

Mary [a fourth student in group 2]: Right, because we had a lot of conversation before we put anything on paper.

Students were reminded that a codification is just a tool and not an end in itself. Even if nothing was drawn on the paper, the paper could still be a stimulus to dialogue. Nevertheless, when we get a code such as this, where the client is pictured as smaller and with less power than the worker, who has little enough power, then the power relations can be problematized. A teacher or worker can ask, "How did it get this way and how can it be changed?"

Mary: The other thing we toyed with was having it more hierarchical, a triangle. There are systems on a smaller scale and larger scale. There are different kinds of power at different times. So what's most pressing or oppressing the client or the social worker at a given time is going to be different from at other times. And that never made it on there.

S1: I was thinking, one way it's good that it wasn't up because it's really all the other systems that go into what makes the DSM-IV. That's what has got to be talked about, not just the manual itself.

S2: Looks like a penis. [great laughter]

Mary: Supposed to be a bomb. [great laughter]

Joe: When we went to draw the picture it became a different discussion.

In this code the client is holding up "all the baggage," including things such as the DSM-IV that they may not even know about. It was suggested that this might be a good codification for workers and clients to talk about together and that workers and clients could create codes collaboratively. A student challenged this last idea. "Just thinking about metaphors. I think, if I were a client, I'd be worried about my life and draw a picture about my house, a kitchen. This is more abstract." We replied that "it certainly could be, unless your kid was in DSS, or you had a court appearance coming up, or you were dealing with a school, or had health issues, or managed care. Then it would be very concrete." Stressed again, however, was the importance of individuals, families, and community groups drawing their own pictures, that is, naming themselves. This would not foreclose a worker/teacher/facilitator commenting on, questioning, or adding to a codification.

Dialogue about a codification can open up many things that are not in the original drawing. For example, the students' lack of knowledge about the history of scholarships for social work education was opened and illuminated as a result of the dialogue about the first code.

Shortly after this discussion, Beth, the presenter from group 3, dealing with the School's summers, described Figure 11.4.

Beth: It's a bridge, not a bed [lots of laughter]. So what we have here is a classroom and it happens to be this classroom where you guys are teaching. Jerry on the left and Fred on the right. You guys are on a bridge. It's what you're trying to do in class. But the context in which this class is happening is the larger context of the School. So there are other issues going on all the time even in this classroom and the stream is supposed to be the dichotomy, the false dichotomy. We had issues that came up in our practice class that were not really dealt with very well. And so on the left we have a student being silenced for thinking some "dangerous thought." On the right, a student, the one who has a blindfold on and doesn't see, is holding that "no poverty" sign with a $60 price tag on it. [laughter in class] And the student down in the bottom corner is saying, "What dichotomy?" and doesn't see any of this going on and those are earmuffs, not a hat. So that was basically it, there is this context going on. There's issues between the students. In this context, where we are trying to bridge the dichotomy in the rest of the School.

F: Questions?
S1: What are Fred and Jerry holding?
S2: Holding hands. [laughter in class]
J: As a clinician I would ask, "What are the dangerous thoughts?"

The students' answers to this question were open and eloquent. They described their fears and the dangers they experienced as they "pretended to create a 'safe' environment to talk about things and bring up issues and go out on a limb." How, "if you don't use or say the right word, you're jumped on and attacked, it's dangerous."

When asked to be more specific, students raised issues of race and culture. "To go against the majority is dangerous. Even if I'm just thinking through an idea out loud that goes against the flow. For example, if one challenged the old format of the racism course [some sections that were white and some that included only people of color] that would be dangerous, because people were angry and upset [that sections would now be integrated]." Class members found

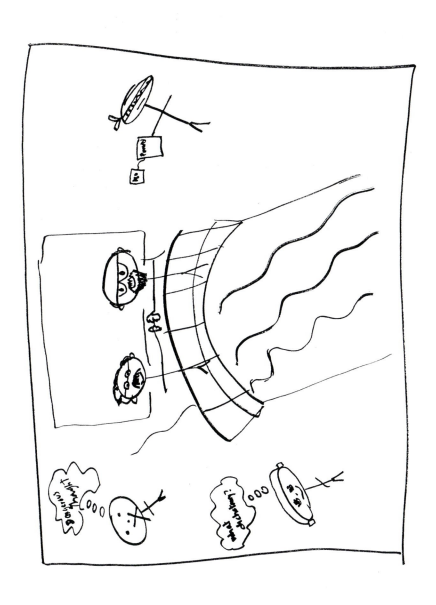

FIGURE 11.4. Dangerous Thoughts

it hard to acknowledge that they "had a lot to learn, and still have a lot to learn. There are a lot of things you have to look at about yourself and it's not always something you want everybody to know."

Students talked about discussions and promises of confidentiality in other classes. We acknowledged their skepticism about this. We do not promise confidentiality, and their bad experiences with confidentiality belie the truth of what is too often promoted. We paraphrase George Simmel (1950) suggesting that "confidentiality can only take place between two people, because then you know who told [laughter in class]." Jerry described how, when a workshop leader asks a group he's in for confidentiality that he, Jerry, says "no," quotes Simmel, and suggests that "like clients who don't know us, it would be unhealthy and diagnostic, if they trust us too quickly." Fred added "You can't mandate and can't artificially create an environment in which people can process honestly and have confidence, an environment in which what they say will be respected rather than attacked. . . . How then do we create an environment in which the ideals that we're describing have a better chance of being enacted?" A student then talked about the illusion of there being a "right answer."

S1: Yeah, with one variable I will skewer the universe. [laughter in class] That's why even this notion of the whole dichotomy, either you're doing social action or clinical social work, because this is what you have to do to make the world a better place yada yada yada. . . . As opposed to them going on simultaneously. To do both is a good thing. You can take a lot of different paths, as opposed to thinking that you have *the* answer.

Another student then made an exceptional point about the history of dialogue. "Dialoguing in traditional forms has meant contending. Argument is the quintessential dialogue. You have to add on to what someone else just said, it's a process." This led to important discussions about struggle, safety, comfort, honesty, good and evil, staying at the table to dialogue, and whether we have the time to work things out.

S1: I think one of the real contradictions is not being honest about what is going on. How are you going to come here and talk about these issues and be comfortable? You can't be comfortable if you're going to talk about certain issues. One does not go with the other. You can't sit down and talk about race and everyone is going to be comfortable, nobody's going to get attacked. So it sets up expectations that are unrealistic to begin with. So people say, "My expectation is I have to feel comfortable, because if I don't, I shut down." And I wonder what the problem is here, and that's not dialogue, and part of the contradiction is having the right expectations. At least you know you are going to feel uncomfortable. You may be attacked. These things will happen here. So the expectation is different when the attacks come. Then we can move forward and then we can actually get to some progress. People have their illusion that you're supposed to feel safe, and, in real dialogue, you're not supposed to feel safe.

S2: That's right.

S3: There's no progress if you feel safe.

F [Relating one of his favorite quotes by Fredrick Douglass]: If there's no struggle there's no progress!

S4: Holding the thought that the people in your classroom basically mean good rather than meaning evil.

S3: If I would say something that you disagree with, you can say "I disagree with that" rather than really going after me. Thinking, at the very least, that I'm a good person, I mean to do well.

J: That is certainly a good wish, but not always true. In this class, on occasion, I'm capable of doing things that are dumb. I'm a whole person, so I do a lot of different things. I'd like to think that if I reflected on the dumb thing and owed someone an apology, that I would give it to them. The question is, will you stay in the room? Not that it's going to be safe in the room, but will you continue to stay in the room, try to work it out? And when we have troubles again, work it out again. And then have more troubles and work it out again. The way things get worked out will change and hopefully the integration of the troubles can take place at a higher level. But, you're in the room and you keep coming back to the room. And sometimes people leave the room for six months, and then come back, because that's part of being human and what dialogue is all about.

At this point a student raised the School's structural dilemma, "Having ten two-hour classes to work things out during a summer semester." Her concern was that this made the consequences for speaking out and saying dangerous things much higher. There was less potential for conflicts to get resolved and "things can end up in a place worse than where you started."

Fred pointed out that the process in dealing with issues of conflict doesn't end in the ten sessions of class. "You need to continue to work on conflicts and recognize that you don't get a neat fantasized closure at the end of ten sessions and sing "Kumbaya." [laughter in class] That ain't going to happen. But, we can continue our own process and process with folks with whom we have conflicts, one on one. We can get three or four people together to deal with issues. There are the limitations to the classroom, but the classroom isn't a boundary to life. And, in life, dialogue can take place."

In the short time that was left before the class ended, students moved between their wish for comfort and safety and their wish to be open and honest and to grow as individuals and as a group. They acknowledged that the world is not always safe. People can be hounded, scapegoated, and fired from jobs for expressing dangerous thoughts. It was also pointed out that almost no one fails a course at Smith for having a dangerous thought.

Fred ended the class with a story about the folksinger Lee Hays of the Weavers. Hays was blacklisted during the McCarthy era. He suffered much isolation and personal pain. He was, however, able to keep his sense of humor and say afterward, "If it wasn't for the honor, I would rather not have gotten blacklisted."

The next class began with time for questions and comments, and then debriefing and expanding the after-class group's discussion of "dangerous thoughts." Some of these "dangerous thoughts" related to the fact that social workers have power. Workers sometimes identify with the elite rather than the people. Students recognized that professionals could use their power in negative ways. Workers may get "secondary gains," such as increased self-esteem, from believing they are "doing good works."

We then brought out a "dangerous thoughts" box which we made that day to much laughter and suggested people could deposit their dangerous thoughts in the box and we would discuss them during the next class. A student quickly, and again to much laughter, noted that "we may need a bigger box."

Creating the dangerous thoughts box acknowledged the hesitancy to raise unpopular opinions around campus, opinions that don't go with the flow. We expressed the hope that the class would leave room for different opinions. We encouraged people to express "dangerous thoughts" and to engage in dialogue. We also connected this with their clinical work. They know thoughts and feelings held back have a way of bubbling up and being displaced in work with clients. The repressed always returns. We suggested that the real test would come in our ability to enact these ideas with each other, not just verbalizing them. Students and clients need to test things out. Testing takes courage and is itself a risk. But testing and passing a test is the way that trust is built:

> That is why, though there may be fear without courage, the fear that devastates and paralyzes us, there may never be courage without fear, that which "speaks" of our humanness as we manage to limit, subject, and control it. (Freire, 1998, p. 41)

We then moved to group 4 and Figure 11.5.

Joyce, the presenter for group 4, interpreted the images in the codification.

Joyce: The person in the middle was representative of us as interns and as students. As you can see, that person looks distressed. What we did was make a pie. Each piece represents different things. That thing in the corner with the words PERSONAL LIFE—NEW IDEAS is a sperm trying to get in. [laughter in class] Basically, the top is representative of Smith: beauty, rainbows, beautiful architecture.

F: So you've got the beauty, and the dove, and the peace sign, the heart, and you've got the college campus.

S1: I think that the beauty is idealized.

FIGURE 11.5. The Life and Worlds of a Student Intern

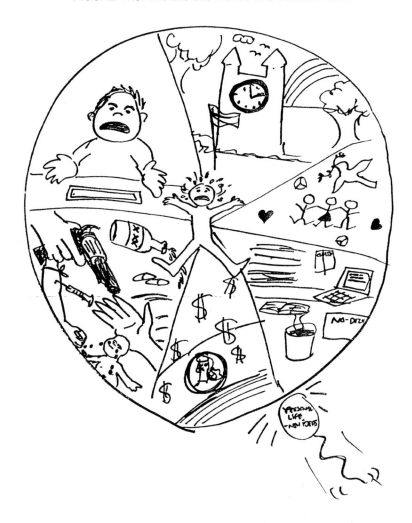

S2: What's that little boy?

Sam [a second student in group 4]: That's a manager or professor, or supervisor. Needs to be fed. Critical and judgmental and wanting, wanting, wanting, wanting from you.

Joyce: Below that is the violence that we see in our work. The stress, there's drug use, the heroin, needles going into an arm, there's a gun. There's a large hand hitting a small child. That's the stuff that we face in the trenches.

S3: What's in the circle with the money piece?

Joyce: How much money it costs to be in this program. Student loans. Living on a shoestring. Next to that is the thesis, homework, and the No-Doz and the laptop with the coffee, and the sperm. We wanted to put out that there are other things trying to break in. We have a personal life trying to break in.

S2: I like the idea that it fertilizes. To bring in new ideas.

S3: What it is trying to do is fertilize the institution.

This codification, like the others, related to the students' stress and the powerlessness they faced in the field. Also present are the demands, including financial demands (it is not unusual for students to finish school with debts that range from $40,000 to $60,000), of different parts of the program. When they dialogued about this, they explored their feelings and experiences about the choices they made and how they might change things, that is, how they might engage in social action.

S1: I don't know if this is a dangerous thought but it struck me that we have a sense of passivity, of things happening to us. I keep coming back to the idea that I chose to come here. I paid the money. If I had a bad time, I'm a sucker. But I come back to that idea that I'm active in this process. Oftentimes the dialogue about what happens to people here is about—it happened to me. I don't know if that's a dangerous thought, but it seems like a tendency to get into a passive stance about things happening to us.

S2: It also speaks to feeling powerless. It's what a lot of people feel like. Whether you have the choice to be here or not. What can you do to change it?

Students responded by saying that it took them three summers to learn they had power and that people would listen.

S3: I've learned that if you really want to change a part of this process you can, but they don't tell you that you can. I've been here two years. I know how much power I could have had over certain parts of the program, but I didn't really exercise that power. I didn't know I could. Now I know. Now I'm leaving.

The instructors pointed out that systems try to maintain a monopoly on what information gets out and at what pace it gets out. When information reaches a student or client or citizen late it is not very useful. Following Marcuse (1965/1976), it was noted that the elite control the media, the source from which the people get information. This prompted a student to observe, "So the elite keeps redefining things. In this case, the people in power at the school are the elite, even though their power in the real world isn't very much."

Students then talked about ways they might try to bring about change. One student suggested that the fourth codification be put on a T-shirt for the next year's orientation as a way to create dialogue with new students. This idea brought the discussion of codifications to a close.

RULES AND SAFETY

In a workshop at the 1998 Bertha Capen Reynolds Society Annual Conference, attended by faculty and students, the idea of rules came up as the way to make a classroom "safe." As workshop leaders, we have no rules with the exception of a rule against any physical violence. This is the only rule we have for our class or for groups we work with in the community. In the workshop we wondered aloud, "Who are the rules for? Who defines and determines what it means to be respectful? Who defines and determines what is hurtful and to whom it is hurtful? Is something hurtful when someone says something 'offensive' or when someone is asked to stuff their feelings, ideas or 'dangerous thoughts'?" As leaders we are not passive bystanders to things that may be hurtful. The level of facilitator activity, when conflict or hurtfulness is in the air, ought to increase dramatically, we believe. The facilitator may move to stand with someone for support, say things that put the heat on himself or herself, use humor, develop role plays, or bring other group members into the process. The work is to facilitate dialogue between group participants, create opportunities for self-reflection, and promote an understanding of the other. In this way, the system is kept open. Indeed, in our experience, rules can shut down the very dialogue that they are ostensibly trying to protect.

Chapter 12

Using Process in Class

Learning and teaching in social work starts with engagement and dialogue. A commitment to dialogical praxis requires that we engage the material presented to us by our clients and begin a process of action and reflection with them. This also applies in the classroom where the clinical content is the work that students bring from the field.

Social work students have grown accustomed to having their work examined in substantial detail by supervisors who require process recording, a "he said/she said" account of a session. In addition, process recordings often include a student's reflections on the work as it proceeds. The supervisor then adds comments and reflections on the process recording and may pick up on parts of the process to engage the student's thinking. The set of dialogues (client/student, student/supervisor, student/teacher) becomes the basis for reflection and learning regarding the work. This phenomenological approach permits going to the "thing itself," the terrain on which the learning takes place.

In class, we ask students to provide copies of process recordings they are willing to share with us and their classmates. Our assumption is that there are potential social action issues are present in every process. All clients and workers live in society and the social institutions of society affect their lives. It would, however, take more time to get to the social action issues in some cases and we are clear that we want to start where a client is. For this reason, we choose processes in which social action issues are relatively transparent and can more quickly be engaged in a way that demonstrates how one might work with them. We do, however, give some time to one or two cases in which connections to social action would need more time. For example, health concerns about her weight brought in by a woman would likely not be engaged immediately as a feminist social action issue. But we would engage why she brought her concern about her weight to a mental health agency. On the other hand, a concern brought in by a woman about sexual harassment on the job might quickly be engaged as a social action issue. We would never, however, want to neglect the way this woman uniquely experiences the harassment.

In class, we applaud the courage of students who are willing to share their work with their fellow students. They take a risk in having that work examined from theoretical and practice perspectives quite different from what they have learned thus far in the program in which we teach. We try to set a tone that is respectful of the work. At the same time, we want to promote thoughtful and critical examination of a student's work with a client. This tone is critical because there is often an element of competitiveness among students. Many students are too quick to point out failings, real and imagined, in the work of others. We want to discourage that practice. We insist that reflection and dialogue be a part of the process, including reflection and dialogue about their competitiveness. Using ourselves as role models, we note that we both have been working for quite a number of years but still need help to recognize places where we make errors in our work. Reflection and dialogue allow us to find ways in which we could have been more useful than we were. As students and as teachers, our work is to learn from our own and others' mistakes. It is in this critical spirit that we hope to examine practice, including our teaching.

We have also found it useful to discuss the concept of "successive approximations," the recognition that over time, both in the longevity of a career and in the life of a clinical relationship, a worker slowly may come closer and closer to "getting it." In this context, "getting it" means both integrating values, theories, and practice and tuning in more effectively to what clients say, feel, and experience. Practice wisdom emerges slowly, over time, and through successive approximations. This awareness allows workers to approach their own practice and the practice of others in an open and humble spirit.

In anticipation of exploring process recordings, a student raised her concern that the class would criticize the work of other students in gratuitously insensitive and harsh ways. Her observation was that students can be "trashed" and that they come away from that experience questioning their ability and their worth as workers. We acknowledged her concern while also suggesting that learning depends on being able to open up one's practice and look at it intensively. We ask people to take responsibility for their critique of one another's work while noting that we will be looking at the process recordings microscopically. To practice from our model, it is necessary to critically examine the work in fine detail and expose the value, theory, and practice assumptions that might interfere with the ability to integrate clinical work and social action.

One year we looked at the work of Ben Williams, a thirty-three-year-old African-American male student, who worked with Frank, a twenty-seven-year-old African-American man. Their work together took place in an urban family service agency that had a sliding fee scale for uninsured clients. Frank was paying the lowest fee on the scale, $5 per session. Ben described Frank's history, including drug and alcohol abuse, drug trafficking, and time in prison. Frank was in a relationship and his girlfriend had recommended that he seek treatment due to problems with impulse control, violence, and homicidal thoughts.

At the time that he began treatment, Frank was working at a local movie theater. During the course of his treatment, there had been an incident at the theater in which a young man was stabbed to death by another young man who attempted to steal the victim's coat. Though Frank did not see the incident, he was in the theater at the time. He also met with the victim's father and was shaken by the episode.

We requested that two people begin a role play as Ben and Frank from the beginning of the process recording that had been distributed in the previous class (see Appendix B). As with any role play, we reserve the option for anyone in the class to stop the action at any point for discussion and dialogue. With this, the role play began.

Frank: Hello, Mr. Williams.
Ben: Hello, Frank.
J: Stop. [Class laughs]

We asked whether there were any questions about the initial greeting.

S1: That "Mr. Williams." Was that agency policy?
Ben: No, that was his thing. He knew my name. That's the way I introduced myself to him the first time and that's what he chose to call me. It wasn't a policy or anything like that.
J: What are the reasons that he would choose that? What interpretations are there about what may have influenced his choice?

The class's responses to this question elicited a wide range of answers. The responses reflected four interrelated areas that need to be considered: clinical, cultural, power/status, and organizational policy considerations.

CLINICAL CONSIDERATIONS

Our students have primarily been trained in psychodynamic models of practice. It was not surprising, therefore, that their first explanation had to do with transference. They wondered whether Frank's calling Ben Mr. Williams had to do with Ben's role as a parental authority figure. Allthough this is possible, they quickly recognized that there was no direct evidence for it. We speculate that their training created an overpsychologized conception of human interactions. It is their world taken for granted.

CULTURAL CONSIDERATIONS

Nancy Boyd-Franklin (1989) discusses the issue of names in relation to family therapy with African-American clients. Her observations are equally relevant in the one-on-one work described here:

> Most therapists spend many years in school, where attitudes and interaction tend to follow along more "casual"' lines than they do in many families. . . . When they begin to join with

families and engage them in family therapy, their natural tendency is to view an informal, "first-name basis" style as putting people at their ease. With Black families, particularly older, more traditional family members, this may be a serious error. The most important lesson here is to take his or her cues from the family. . . . It is usually helpful to start with a more formal introduction and allow the family to indicate their preference. (pp. 109-110)

The fact that both the worker and the client were African-American men is significant in this case. This issue is discussed by Boyd-Franklin (1989) when she observes:

The Black male therapist may be perceived as a professional, less street wise, and so on. There may even be suspicions about the therapist's masculinity because he does not assume a more traditional Black male role. An important aspect of the credibility that the Black male therapist must establish in these situations is that of establishing himself as a peer. (p. 104)

The fact that client and worker are not peers, however, is obvious to both of them. The client's use of the title Mr. in addressing his worker is a subtle, or perhaps direct, statement of his recognition of that difference. While these issues also include concerns about power and status, it must be recognized that power and status are themselves greatly influenced by culture.

At the same time, some students speculated that Frank's calling Ben Mr. Williams could be a sign of respect. It was seen by some of the students and by the worker himself as, at least in part, reflecting recognition of Ben's achievement in attaining a professional role in service to the community.

It was apparent from the material that Frank felt comfortable calling Ben Mr. Williams. Ben reported that Frank preferred to be called Frank. The way they agreed to address each other appears, on the surface, to be respectful culturally. However, it needs to be recognized that the historical development of African-American culture took place in a highly politicized atmosphere. As Paulo Freire has noted, the ability to name oneself is always political.

POWER/STATUS CONSIDERATIONS

Another interpretation of the interchange between Ben and Frank relates to their relative power and status. One student noted: "Though they are both African-American men, they are not peers." In community mental health agencies, clients tend to have less power and are of lower status than clinicians.

This difference in power and status can impede dialogue whether or not it is intentionally or consciously imposed. We asked how this related to the clinical encounter between Ben and Frank. Ben himself responded, "Well, the theme throughout his life seemed to be that he was always in the system, he was always powerless." Frank's powerlessness was then connected to the theme of violence. We wondered how much the interchange around naming reflected the two participants' culture and how much it reflected the violence embedded in the power differentials of the mental health system.

We suggested that it would be worthwhile to problematize dialogue with Frank about why he chose to call the worker Mr. Williams. Through this dialogue, the worker might get Frank's interpretation and not be limited to his own. Similarly, it would be critical for the worker to reflect on how he came to call his client by his first name, reinforcing the power and status differences already present in the system.

The instructors then moved the class back to the role play in an attempt to demonstrate how the above issues could be engaged.

J: OK, let me suggest a way that I might do it. Let's role-play a little here.

J [playing Ben]: When you first came in, I called you Frank and you called me Mr. Williams, and you just did it again and I'm just wondering . . . [long silence]

Ben [playing Frank]: I don't know. That's what your name is. That's what they said who I'll be seeing, so that's what I call you.

J: You'll be seeing Mr. Williams?

B: Yeah.

J: Now, you know my name is Ben Williams . . . ? [long silence]

B: OK, I think that's what to call you. It's what I call my parole officer if I go see him.

J: And you'd like me to call you . . . ?

B: Frank.

J: Frank?

B: You call me Frank.

J: What about that? You call me Mr. Williams and I call you Frank?

B: I'm not sure what you're asking.

J: That's a good place to start and I'm glad you said you're not sure. I'm calling you by your first name and you're calling me by my last name. And I'm just wondering about that. And I also wonder whether it has to do in any way with what we've been talking about for a couple of minutes. You know, about controlling yourself?

B: XXX

J: And yet you'd like me to call you by your first name?

B: I'm not used to being called by my last name unless I'm in court or unless I'm in trouble or something.

J: So this is like court or you're in trouble?

B: No.

J: Oh, the other way around?

B: I'm not used to people addressing me formally, by my last name, unless I'm in trouble.

J: Unless you're in trouble? So I misunderstood. Sorry. [Here the meaning of informality was missed]

The role play revealed the recognition that titles and names have intrapersonal, interpersonal, cultural, and political meanings. There was little wish on Frank's part (in this role play) to explore those meanings more deeply. At this stage, the worker would move on to other elements of the material that Frank brings into the treatment process. But, and this is central to dialogical praxis, the issue has been engaged, themes have surfaced, and the dialogue can be revisited as these themes resurface in the course of the work. The response may be different at those times.

ORGANIZATIONAL POLICY CONSIDERATIONS

The range of experiences students had in their agencies, related to policies regarding how they and their clients would address each other, was quite broad. At one end of the continuum, some agencies required that both worker and client be called by their last names. At the other end, workers and clients were free to find their own ways of naming themselves and each other. Despite these differences in policies, there was a common pattern in practice that replicated Frank and Ben's experience. Specifically, workers were generally accorded a formal title and clients were called by their first names. This was particularly true when clinical, cultural, and power/status issues were more prominent in a given agency setting.

SOME ADDITIONAL REFLECTIONS: NAMES, TITLES, AND TIMING

When we raised the issue of names by stopping the role play after the first lines, students reacted with some consternation and impatience. There was a sense that raising the name issue at this stage was "artificial." The question of artificiality would, on the surface, appear to have some merit. Frank did not explicitly raise the question, "How come I have to call you Mr. Williams and you call me Frank?" Our values call for a worker to wait for the client to raise issues, not for workers to come in with their own agenda.

Yet, we also are committed to dialogical praxis. Interactions and issues can be problematized. Only in this way can a worker see whether a client is ready to engage with and explore issues and phenomena that have been raised, however implicitly. It would be inappropriate to raise an issue and then compel the client to stick with it against his or her wishes, even if that were possible. As clinicians, however, we would still want to engage clients' resistance or defensiveness to gain an understanding of what prevented their willingness to explore with us an issue that they implicitly raised.

In this sense, the question is not so much one of artificiality but one of when and how to intervene in an issue that is existentially present but has not been explicitly raised by the client. It is an issue of timing.

In the current example, the instructors, while agreeing that the timing in the role play was off, still wanted to underline the issue. However artificial this was, the class did observe that the issue existed implicitly and needed, at some point, to be addressed and engaged. It was suggested that the way to engagement might be a metaphor Frank opened, or a comment Frank might make about names in another context.

It was acknowledged that starting off with the first two sentences of a process recording from a particular session loaded the dice. But, an instructor noted, "That's where we started because that's where Ben and Frank started. Had we gone further down into the process and picked up something else, we'd be off on a different tangent with some different artificiality. What we hope for is that we can take a piece of work and look at it under a microscope and see the tremendous variety of issues there are and the many ways one can work with those issues. At best, through successive approximations, the most appropriate issue is engaged at the most appropriate time."

The point was made that this is no different than beginning any therapeutic work. Students were reminded how "artificial" it was and how uncomfortable they felt the first time they met a client or dealt with a new issue such as drinking or sexual abuse. It was suggested that there is a good reason we call what we do *practice* and that therapeutic work, talking about things one would not dream of engaging in other contexts, becomes "natural" as a result of practice.

After this, a student did thoughtfully remind us that what becomes natural for us may not be natural for the client. "I think it's important not to lose the perspective of somebody who hasn't come from twenty years of analysis and comes into your office."

Another student added to this. "I just want to say one thing about that interaction that you had. When you said, 'You call me Mr. Williams and I call you Frank' and then were silent. That silence was excruciating. I don't know if anyone else felt that way when that happened. The need to let a client sit when that happens. It's hard."

The instructors then summarized and suggested that the discussion of names and how they were used had connections to other issues that were soon to come up in the process. Indeed, everything Frank (or any other client) raises is connected to the clients themselves and, therefore, those things are connected to each other.

VIOLENCE

A central issue in the discussion of naming was the issue of power differentials and status. During the discussion of power, the theme of violence quickly emerged. In its broadest sense, they understood that Frank's poverty and lack of power, in the process of naming, could be seen as examples of violence. The entire structure of the therapeutic process, particularly when it is mandated, may well be seen as coercive and violent. Violence is embedded in the historic social control function of social work and the other "helping" professions.

Some might still question whether what we described above could truly be called violence. There was no ambiguity, however, about whether to use that term to describe the murder that Frank reported in his work with Ben. For much of the remainder of this chapter, and in the next, we focus on issues related to violence in Frank's life and in the broader community.

To get at this material and to bridge the dichotomy between clinical work and social action, students were asked to divide into four groups and develop a role play focused on that part of the process in which Frank described the killing at the movie theater. We specifically directed them to that part of the process (see Appendix B) where the worker asks Frank, "So how is the job going?" The task of each group was to examine the process and decide how they might intervene. We asked them to develop an approach that took into account the personal while connecting it to social action work. This approach needed to be grounded in something Frank talked about during the session. Our instructions to the students were to identify an issue that was not only a personal phenomenon for Frank but also, in C. Wright Mills' terms, a social problem. For good clinical work to take place they need to be connected. When the students returned from their groups, a student began by talking about her group's discussion.

S1: I'm really glad we got to this because this is why I took the class. It's so hard to bring in these larger issues when you're talking to someone in a therapeutic situation, and that's what we are grappling with. We are trying to figure out how to say that stuff. If you want to bring in these larger issues you want to let that person know that they are not the only person that this is happening to, that they are not at fault. It's a social problem.

This said, the students, playing the worker and client, began the role play.

Worker: After I asked who stabbed him, that's where we start.

Client: I don't know who the guy was, but he wanted his coat and the kid told him he can have it but he stabbed the kid anyway. It kind of shook me up. . . . It made me cry . . . I've been a little disturbed about it lately.

Worker [moving away from the text]: So, I'm wondering, what are your thoughts about the stabbing?

Client: Maybe it has something to do with respect or something, like he wasn't getting any respect or he needed to get control. It happens all the time.

Worker: What happens?

Client: Everywhere around me in this community, people are always hitting each other and stabbing each other and it all has to do with, if you wanted something, wanted a coat, but also feeling that you don't have anything.

Worker: I'm confused. He could have gotten the coat without violence but he chose to stab him in spite of that.

Client: He really wanted to prove something. I know what that feels like. I've done that myself.

Worker: So you say you felt bad? Tell me.

Client: Well, I guess I just got mad. I feel like I didn't have anything, that I didn't have any money, that I didn't even have anybody looking at me like I was worth anything. So it just made me so furious. I just wanted to do something and I just wanted to hurt people.

Worker: So, do you find that's a problem in your community?

In this role play, the students, we think too abruptly, connected the violence in Frank's personal life to the violence in his community.

A bit later in the role play, the student playing Frank offered that, "It makes me feel powerful, it makes me feel like I have control over something. I mean, I don't have any money; we don't have any businesses; we don't have any way to get anything. So it makes me feel less passive, like I can make the other person feel even weaker that I am. He's lying there on the ground. At least I'm not." Here the client's experience of passivity and lack of control in relation to the world of money and privilege is perceived by him as violence. The individual's violence in this context is a way to gain control and respect and to counter the violence is experienced from the larger society.

Despite the truth of the above generalization, the central question in the class related to this role play was whether this was the best place to bridge the false dichotomy between "typical" clinical work and social action. The jump to address the community was seen as premature by the instructors and most students. In our model, we believe that we must stay where the client is. Frank's personal issues would need to be engaged first, his pain, tears, nervousness, and "shook-upness" related to the murder and his meeting with the victim's father.

There was, however, a very direct opportunity to bridge the dichotomy between clinical work and social action later in the session. Specifically, Frank said, "I try to talk to the young 'uns at work . . . they be talking about stealing cars and selling drugs. I be telling them stories about the things I did and what happened to me. I tell them I know it's all fun now but it's not worth it in the long run." The instructor noted that Frank, "when he describes himself talking to the kids, was on the verge of doing community action without us." (Laughter.) From here it would be a short step to ask Frank, "What else might be done to engage the young 'uns?" This topic will be explored more fully in the next chapter.

Again, it was pointed out that one always works with successive approximations. Nobody gets it exactly right. No matter how much experience you have, the best one can do is to find a "good enough" place to engage. The more experience one has, the greater the comfort and the better one gets at picking the right place to intervene. This practice wisdom is partly unconscious and, over time, becomes less artificial.

The discomfort students or workers have addressing and engaging social action possibilities that clients bring to treatment may not only be related to their inexperience. It also has to do with the anxiety they have about the real and imagined dangers of doing so.

However much there is a hook in reality, some of this anxiety may be defensive. To engage the violence that emerges from the political and economic disempowerment of the African-American community would entail a number of risks. On a personal level, workers, and especially white workers, would have to examine or come to terms with their own privilege, powerlessness, and inaction. On an agency level, workers who raise issues of race as it affects agency policies and practices risk losing status and jobs. On a political level, workers who are willing to challenge racism face the risks of labeling, stigma, physical violence, and even death.

REFLECTIONS ON RACE

Emerging from a role play developed by another group was a discussion about the reality that Ben and Frank were both African-American men. This had meaning for the work. In this role play, Frank said to Ben, "You know what I mean," referring to the ways in which African Americans are treated. It was pointed out that when a client directly addresses a worker, the only other person in the room, this comment must be engaged. In this role play, the client offered a direct invitation to interact Subject-to-Subject. The question for the worker was whether to accept the invitation. The real Ben, who responded to this role play, was conflicted. Specifically, he was concerned that fully taking up Frank's invitation and moving with him into social action would compromise the therapeutic work. His concern was about how to engage the "social action piece but stay within the confines of the therapeutic process."

In this instance, to accept Frank's invitation would be to recognize that both worker and client are African-American men, that Ben and Frank share a common racial status in the larger society. This recognition has the potential for creating a different level of dialogue between them. Subject-to-Subject dialogue would be less caught up in the names and roles that were assigned to them by the agency. Subject-to-Subject relationships still have different therapeutic roles. They contain two unique individuals who have been socialized differently and may have come from very different communities. But the power relationship has shifted in a way that makes dialogical praxis possible.

Chapter 13

Taking the Work to the Community

In the previous chapter, the classroom focus was on helping students see that there was a place where they could begin working toward a simultaneous focus on clinical work and social action. The violence in Frank's community was the issue chosen to do this. Frank had already begun this work on his own by talking to young people in the community about the toll that violence was taking on all of them.

The work being done by Frank and Ben has, thus far, been dyadic. To bridge the false dichotomy, interventions need to move beyond the dyad to the social-structural level. This chapter's focus will be on how the class took the work to the agency and the community.

Our discussion will describe how the class moved to social action in the agency and the community. We will present the process of the class and also comment on that process. Moving to the agency and to the community will involve more actors and, necessarily, create greater complexity. It stretches the boundaries of clinical work but it does not change the fact that the work continues to be clinical. Like clinical work, social action work is a slow and arduous process.

The next step was to expand the discussion between Ben and Frank about Frank's speaking to young people about the violence in the community. How would Ben begin to play a role in addressing it? In a role play, Ben asked how Frank might proceed with his wish to reach the young people in the community.

Frank: I don't know what I would do about it.
Ben: That is a good place to start. I don't know—a good way to start. Are there other people that you know in the community to talk about it with?

F: Yes, they don't know what to do about it either. So you just find out about it and you have to survive. Just one guy can't do anything.

B: That's true.

F: One guy doesn't have power.

B: That's true, too. If there's just one guy, you can't do almost anything. So, is it possible to get a bunch of different guys and gals together?

F: To do what?

B: That's a good question. We can all start from the place that we are at. We don't know.

F: What would you do?

B: We can talk about it together.

F: I talk to people on the street. It doesn't make it any better. We just talk about how we feel about it and so we are just talking.

B: Do you feel better when you talk?

F: Well, it's better than not.

B: That is the place to start off.

F: We can't do anything about it.

B: I don't know if we can or we can't. But I think you are right about one thing you can't do it alone. What I am putting out to you—I don't know if you have an interest in it at all—is to get some folks who you talk to together and they might talk about it together here. I'd be glad to talk with you.

F: What's the use of talking about it? A guy gets killed.

B: That was a terrible thing.

F: And he ultimately didn't do anything.

B: I would be more than glad to meet with the folks that you talked about. And some other folks could be brought in.

Described in the above is Ben's offer to work with Frank at a new level, in the community. Why would Frank jump into this? Frank has his own concerns, without trying to change the world. And he would have to vouch for Ben, someone he really doesn't know personally, with the young people. He is also being asked to trust that the agency will play a supportive role in dealing with the violence being played out in the community. For Frank to take Ben up on his offer, a solid relationship of trust would have to exist.

Trust began to develop in the process of Frank's testing Ben about his blackness. This was played out in several role plays. In one role play, Frank asks Ben, "You know what I mean?," referring to ways in which they, as African Americans, are treated. In another role play, Frank refers to the practice of "white cops" pulling over cars driven by African-American men and asks, "You've been through some of this, haven't you?" In response to these questions, the instructors suggested the need to respond directly and affirmatively. The worker is black, reads the paper, has had negative experiences being black, and knows that terrible things happen to black people in the community. By identifying with his and Frank's blackness, a relationship and a working alliance could be built between them.

This alliance was, however, only part of the equation necessary to begin to do social action work. The other half of the equation is the agency. Before Frank can be asked to engage his friends or other members of the community, the agency's commitment to be part of the process must be secured. Students raised questions about whether the agency could or would buy into this new mode of working. They raised questions about funding issues and political concerns. Their questions were both legitimate and a sign of the resistance they had to this type of work. This opened a dialogue in the classroom about how we would respond to these concerns and deal with the agency.

Specifically, we acknowledged that there are risks to an agency that moves in this direction. There is also the potential for positive outcomes. Although it is unlikely that any current funding could easily be used for this work, new funding sources targeted at violence prevention or community building, as examples, could be cultivated. Similarly, there could be some political cost for "rocking the boat," but there is also the potential for the agency to create new political alliances. In addition, work of this sort probably is consistent with the agency's mission statement, which, like those of most agencies, includes serving the community. Not to engage in violence prevention would put the agency in a contradiction. These strategies for overcoming agency resistance are examples of a concept we playfully call "wiggle room."

Wiggle room is that space between an organization's rigid refusal to act in a particular way or engage an issue and the possibility that there may be room to do so. It starts from the assumption that nothing is set in stone, that through creativity the worker can find the wiggle room to move the organization in a desired direction. For example, there are often allies among the staff. There may be a sympathetic board member or community leader who could be helpful. A supportive faculty field supervisor from the school might provide some leverage. Finally, the supervisor and agency managers can be helped to act on their idealism and ethical principles. Too often, these are lost in the day-to-day pressures of running an organization.

Although working with wiggle room might push the agency boundaries and make people uncomfortable, it would not violate any agency rules, and it would keep the dialogue going. It is critical, in this context, to point out that workers who push agency boundaries and make people uncomfortable have to be above reproach in all other areas of agency life. They must come to work and meetings on time, get their paperwork in promptly, participate in agency functions, and, generally, provide no opportunity for administration to discipline them over minor issues. They need to be good citizens.

We distinguish between wiggle room and what we call an "end run." Wiggle room operates within agency policies and mandates and attempts to use multiple internal remedies out of a commitment to dialogical praxis. End runs, on the other hand, may violate or sabotage agency rules and are antidialogical. In end runs, workers "freelance," and they rationalize their behavior as a "higher good" justified by their belief that the organization is incapable of change. They do not understand or respect the potential negative consequences of their actions. For example, going to a funder about organizational behavior that a worker believes to be unethical, without attempting to dialogue, fully understand, and remedy the situation internally, could jeopardize jobs, the agency's survival, and, most important, services to clients.

To involve the agency, the next step is to engage the supervisor. We set up a role play using a "fishbowl" structure to explore the obstacles we could anticipate and strategies to overcome them. In the fishbowl format, all the action takes place in the center of the room and observers are free to substitute themselves for one of the actors.

We structure the exercise in the following way. We start from the assumption that, in addition to Ben and the supervisor, there are other unacknowledged actors in the room. For example, the agency board and executive director are strong influences on anything the supervisor might say. Frank and the community are influences on Ben. We literally give voice to these actors by having students playing these roles stand behind Ben and the supervisor. This is done to make explicit the conflicting forces influencing the dialogue. For example, if the supervisor seems too agreeable to this unconventional approach, the student playing the agency might express concern about possible public relations problems that could result. Similarly, if Ben is too concerned about the agency's perspective, the student playing Frank might say something such as, "Don't forget about the community." In essence, they are the personification of the multiple voices influencing us in our interactions.

In preparing for the role play, students are asked to tune in to the ways in which the supervisor is likely to respond. This means tuning in to the supervisor's educational and administrative functions. In addition, a particular supervisor's self-interest must be taken into account. The educational role is grounded in the expectation that the supervisor teaches practice and accepts the responsibility to help a student develop professional skills and attitudes. In their administrative roles, supervisors must consider how a student's work will affect the agency and how the agency would want that supervisor to respond. Beyond this, supervisors have their personal self-interests, including how a student's actions will affect their status, salary, and even continued employment. The strategies that are developed should flow from the assessment of how these influences affect the supervisor.

A student's strategic use of process recordings is one way to respond to the supervisor's educational role. In this case, Ben's reflective writing on the previous session with Frank could raise the question of violence in the community, its impact on Frank, and Frank's desire to play a role in engaging the youth of the community. It would also raise Ben's involvement in the process.

In response to the administrative role, a student could suggest the availability of funds for crime prevention and community building. In addition, he could point out how the agency could increase its status by playing a visible leadership role in a vital community issue.

Any supervisor would have to see and believe that whatever action took place would not harm her or his interests and might even be a benefit. For example, the supervisor's concern about public image and fund-raising opportunities could be seen by the agency executive as a demonstration of management potential.

Presuming that our strategies for influencing the supervisor have worked, the next step would be to arrange for a presentation by Frank, Ben, and the supervisor to a management meeting at the agency. Though it is unconventional to bring a client to a management meeting, our values related to self-determination and dialogue demand it. In addition, there is some potential strategic advantage in having a community member be part of a request to the agency to play an active role on a community issue. It might be uncomfortable for an agency's leadership to say no to a community member on such an important issue.

For the purposes of the class, we assume that the arguments the supervisor found persuasive would also be appealing to the agency's management. It was agreed that the agency would take leadership in convening a community meeting on violence. Students are helped to recognize that, with new actors, there will be additional agendas and interests at play. This is a complicated process and it should not be simplified. The agency's interests and methods may not always coincide with those of the grassroots community, business leaders, church leaders, and so on. For example, an inevitable consequence of the agency's agreement to convene the meeting is that it will determine the invitation list and agenda. As much as possible, a worker practicing from our model will continue to push for Frank and other grassroots community members to be involved in the planning and implementation of the community meeting.

Having established that there will be a community meeting, the next step is to strategize about who should attend. Toward that end, we engaged the class in a brainstorming session.

F: We thought it would be useful to begin to think collectively about who ought to be at the table. Who are the people and interests that ought to be in coalition that can have some impact on the degree of violence in the community? This is not just going to happen because a bunch of social workers sit around talking. There are players in the community that would need to be brought into the mix. So who should be there?

S1: Members of the community.

F: Members of the community. Can you be more specific?

S2: People affected by the violence.

S3: Could we get someone like the father of that kid who got killed?

J: That would be really powerful. Who else?

S4: Social service providers?

S5: Some of Frank's friends.

It is important that Frank's friends be part of the first community meeting. Their presence confers legitimacy on them and their concerns. It is essential that people with little power be a part of the process from the beginning. Coalitions typically do not get much broader than they are at the first meeting. This point is especially relevant when marginalized people are invited later in the process. They rightly see the belated reaching out as treating them as an afterthought.

S6: How about the police?

J: Interesting choice, but we need to understand that having the police and Frank's friends in the room at the same time may create some tension. Work will have to be done in advance with both groups in order to help them work together. It needs to be recognized that both bring some baggage to the table with them.

S7: How about the newspapers?

This is the first place where a strategic decision had to be made about inclusion or exclusion. One consideration is the role of the press. Newspapers are there to report. Reporters are not necessarily allies. Strategic planning about when to let them in and when to keep them out is important. You need to have confidence that people in the room are not going to be fighting with one another when the press is there. You need to know who the reporter will be. There are reporters on every paper who specialize in different beats. If it is possible, a reporter who is community oriented and would be sympathetic to the community being mobilized against violence should be invited.

Frank asked, "Who else needs to be there?" Students suggested that representatives of the clergy, the schools, the local political structure, and businesspeople all need to be represented. More than one clergyperson should be invited because there are often political dynamics among the religious institutions within a community. One approach is to invite the leadership of the local ministerial alliance or interfaith council. In addition, there are other groups of significant clergy who do not participate in interfaith groups, or particularly powerful church leaders who would need to be invited.

Dealing with youth violence requires cooperation with the schools. Key leaders from the school system, such as principals, PTA officials, and school board members, would need to be invited.

Decisions about which politicians to invite and what the planning committee hopes to get from their presence have tactical and strategic implications. For example, an elected official who was sympathetic could lend legitimacy and support to the group. On the other hand, an unsympathetic official could provide a target for future organizing. The fact that a politician will use a meeting of community leaders for his or her own political agenda and inhibit dialogue is always a concern.

To build a broad coalition, businesspeople need to be invited. They bring respectability, access to political and economic power, and, in this instance, have a stake in reducing the violence that keeps people away from the downtown commercial district.

An important consideration in planning the first community meeting is the size of the group. It needs to be large enough to establish legitimacy, seriousness, and the breadth of community concern. At the same time, it cannot be so large as to be unmanageable.

In this light, who facilitates the meeting will be crucial. It is virtually certain that the executive director of Ben's agency will assume that role. Very few executives are willing to have a meeting at their agency with elected officials, the press, and community leaders present without playing the lead role. The exception to this could be a situation in which someone from the community is so widely viewed as a community leader that it would be unseemly to usurp that person's acknowledged role.

In addition, it is useful to assign specific roles to particular meeting attendees. For example, a member of the clergy would be asked to provide a religious invocation. In this meeting, the father of the murder victim might be asked to offer some opening remarks. Finally, given that they brought the issue to the agency's attention, Frank and Ben should be asked to provide background on how the meeting came to be.

Several things worth talking about surfaced in the role play of the meeting. We have already noted the tensions that likely exist between the young people Frank brought to the meeting and the police. In the role play, the meeting became a place for them to talk about their differences. In an ongoing dialogue, the police could come to see the young people as human beings and the young people might gain a greater appreciation for the role of the police. For this to happen, the meeting facilitator would need to take an active role and clearly articulate the tensions between these two groups. Only in this way could progress toward resolution take place.

A second tension that occurred in the role play revolved around the elected official's use of the meeting as a political platform. The facilitator would need to find a way to manage the politician's need to be heard at the expense of the meeting's agenda.

It was also recognized that there would be differences in attendees' education, status, experience, and comfort in participating in formal meetings. This might be the first meeting of this sort that the young people Frank invited ever attended. The leader would need to be understanding and respectful and facilitate their participation as equals in the meeting.

If it is to be the catalyst for a positive community response to violence, this meeting must be the first of several. Before people leave, a date and agenda for the next meeting needs to be set. In addition, attendees should have some assignment to be accomplished between meetings. For example, the PTA and clergy representatives might be asked to go back to their constituents and see what receptivity there is to participating in a community antiviolence effort. They also should be asked to solicit ideas to bring to the next meeting. Finally, additional community representatives may need to be invited to the next meeting.

The previouse suggestions and approaches were part of the post-role play debriefing done by the class. They represent only a small part of what would go into organizing a campaign such as the one envisioned here. (See Bobo, Kendall, and Max, 1991, for material on organizing a campaign.)

After the meeting, clinical work with Frank continues. Ben needs to dialogue with him about his experience at the meeting. He might be ambivalent, and this ambivalence would need to be explored. For example, he might feel proud that he helped to initiate the meeting but angry that he did not play a large leadership role. In this case, the meeting becomes a parameter (Eissler, 1953) in the clinical work.

In our model, there is no discontinuity between clinical work and social action. One constantly flows into and enriches the other. There is no dichotomy.

Chapter 14

The Course Assignment

The first time we taught this class, the primary assignment was a paper due at the last class. This withdrawal from the "bank," the students' heads, where we had "deposited knowledge," left little room for dialogue about the paper itself. Students had no chance to share the insights, issues, questions, or misunderstandings they had about the concepts and ideas they wrote about. The following year, after our own reflection and dialogue, we divided the paper into three parts (see Paper Assignment, p. 188). This new format allows students to get quick feedback and creates the opportunity for dialogue. It allows the instructors to bring students' ideas, feelings, and practice into the class for discussion and reflection.

The paper's primary function is for students to think analytically, strategically, and dialogically about contradictions related to their practice. The format has also uncovered clinical issues, organizational issues, and other questions and concerns that can be addressed in class. The instructors get an idea of where students are and have examples of work students have written from the students' perspective. This work can be problematized as well as used as a role model for other students.

In the introduction to the assignment, students are informed that both instructors read each paper and will make comments and suggestions about how students might approach the next section of the paper. Students also find that the instructors regularly make comments about each other's comments, agreeing, expanding, disagreeing, or just having fun. This helps set a serious and playful tone for the paper and the class. Students are not asked to rewrite previous parts of the paper, but are asked to respond to comments and include the reasons they may have changed the paper's direction.

PAPER ASSIGNMENT

The assignment is one paper to be submitted in three installments. This will allow us to provide you with feedback and have dialogue in class as part of the process of developing the paper. We encourage you to incorporate our comments into each subsequent submission. It is not necessary to redo the previous submission.

Reflect on your practice with a client(s) during your internship.

PART A: (1) What were the contradictions you experienced? Be explicit and present clear, detailed examples of these contradictions in practice.

(2) What are the psychosocial structural factors that underlie these contradictions? Again, you need to be explicit and clearly explicate these factors at the personal, agency, professional, and social institutional level.

DUE: Third Session

PART B: Understanding the above, how might you change your practice to resolve these contradictions? Give clear, explicit examples of what you would do and say.

DUE: Sixth Session

PART C: Finally, what consequences and reactions could you anticipate from clients, supervisors, the School, agency, community, yourself, and/or other relevant audiences to your new action?

DUE: Ninth Session

The remainder of this chapter explores, following the outline of the paper, selected case examples of the contradictions students experienced in their practice, how students understood these contradictions, the students' speculations about how these contradictions might have been engaged and resolved, and the consequences they believed might result from this new engagement. In addition, ideas, concerns, issues, and questions that emerged from the paper assignment are discussed and analyzed. We again thank our students for their courage and generosity in giving us permission to use their work.

INTRODUCTION TO CASES

Workers who subscribe to the values in our model are in a contradiction when their behavior is in conflict with the interrelated core values of self-determination, economic and political justice, and a commitment to dialogical praxis. Professionals who do not subscribe to the values essential to our model are in contradiction when their practice is in conflict with the values embedded in their professional codes of ethics or with their personal values. An agency is in contradiction when its operations and procedures, informal or formal, conflict with its mission statement and/or stated policies.

CASE # 1: CONTRADICTION RELATED TO SELF-DETERMINATION

In part A, Marie, the student, described her placement in a special education program that was connected to a psychiatric hospital in a large city in the Midwest. One of her assignments was to work with Toni, a thirteen-year-old girl, and her poor, ethnic Catholic family, who had lived with their modified extended family (Litwak, 1960) in the city for several generations. Toni's involvement in the special education program related to her difficulties in reading. There were also concerns about her behavior, including glue sniffing, staying out past curfew, leaving home without permission, and possible prostitution. Toni and her family (mother, stepfather, and four siblings) were involved with the police, probation, the Department of Juvenile Justice, the Department of Social Services (DSS), and a variety of other agencies.

In this agency, all families were required to see a worker in order for their child to attend the hospital's special education program.

The program's "philosophy . . . was that for treatment to be effective, the family system must be involved." Marie reported that other members of the treatment team would have wanted Toni's parents to take the initiative and make plans for their children. On the surface, the agency and its professionals were committed to the value of self-determination. Marie as well was personally and professionally committed to the value of "self-determination, with the goal that clients be allowed to act on their own initiative."

In spite of the commitment to self-determination by Marie's agency, other professionals working with the case, and Marie herself, the day-to-day work with Toni and her family was filled with contradictions. For example, team meetings and meetings with other agencies excluded Toni and her family. Marie reported that she became, with the encouragement of her supervisor, overinvolved in decision making, including exploring the possibility of removing Toni from her family and placing her in a therapeutic group home.

The intrapersonal, interpersonal, and social forces that created contradictions with the value of self-determination are well illustrated in this case. For example, Marie wanted to be "helpful and important." She reported her own need to "exercise agency" even if it turned out to be "at the family's expense." She noted that there was both pressure and support from her treatment team, supervisor, and professionals from other agencies "to do something," to "fix" things. Finally, the family, and especially Toni's overburdened mother, saw Marie "as the expert and would ask for advice and decision making."

The fact that the violation of self-determination was not seen or felt consciously as a contradiction by Marie and her co-workers during her work with Toni and her family, needs to be explained. What allows self-determination to be terminated?

In this case, the family's status was degraded (Garfinkle, 1956). Successful degradation, according to Garfinkle, requires that the family be labeled by legitimate agents, such as professional workers from social agencies. The professionals working with Toni's family used the labels "dysfunctional" and "unsafe" in this "degradation ceremony" (Garfinkle, 1956). By these measures, the family was not worthy and did not have the right to self-determination. This

family's poverty, lack of education, and powerlessness also contrib-
uted to the denial of self-determination as a value in practice. The
family was stigmatized as "unworthy." Their involvement did not
have to be considered. Finally, Marie's feelings of helpfulness as a
worker and her wish to be a good student who would be labeled
"diligent and caring" conspired with the family's, and particularly
Toni's mother's, needs and fatalism to abrogate self-determination.

To be comfortable with the contradiction between one's values
and behavior, professional workers, with the help of supervisors,
colleagues, and sometimes clients, find ways to rationalize their
behavior. Ways are found to change the formulation of what is
"right" and "good" work. Ways are found to defend against the
experience of living in a contradiction. Ways are found to define
controlling behavior as a higher good.

In part B of her paper, Marie suggested three ways she might
have changed her behavior to resolve the contradiction related to
self-determination. First, she would do home visits. This was, in
fact, the family's preference. It would relieve them of issues related
to child care and transportation. Appointments could be kept and
more members of the family could be involved. Extended family
and close friends who might provide support and help in opening
decision-making possibilities could be included.

Second, Marie would involve the family, and particularly Toni's
mother, in the referral process. This assumes they had an interest in
finding a group home where Toni might stay for a time. This would
give the family an active role and involve them in any plans that
were developed.

The third change would be to include family members, particularly Toni's mother, in meetings Marie had with other agencies and
in team meetings. What was observed in these new intervention
strategies was Marie's attempt to engage in dialogical praxis with
Toni and her family. This praxis will increase the possibility of their
becoming self-determining in decisions that affect their lives.

In part C of the paper, Marie explored the reactions of different
audiences to her new intervention strategy. She believed that the
family would welcome the home visits since they made the family's
life easier. On the other hand, the agency might not be so welcoming. Its policy was to have families come to the agency. Marie also

described her supervisor as "trying to help me adopt a new identity as a family therapist, which meant I was supposed to give up home visits." One of the instructors ironically noted in a side comment that social workers started out as friendly visitors and for many families, such as Toni's, this agency should itself be labeled "hard to reach."

Marie believed that her supervisor would see involving Toni's family in the process of referral to a group home as good work, as helping the family to get more involved. Resistance would more likely come from the group home, which required a "professional referral." Toni's mother, whose socialization did not include dealings with formal organizations, might also be resistant. In addition, Marie insightfully recognized that by making the referral herself, Toni's mother would be spared the ambivalence and guilt she had about the possibility of giving up and rejecting her daughter. This intrapsychic issue would need to be engaged as part of the process if Toni's mother were to take on a more self-determining stance. Marie believed that the possibility of one or a few family members attending team meetings or interagency meetings "would be met with a flat 'no.' "

Finally, Marie recognized that she had her own internal work to do. She would need to get over the idea that doing things for this family made her helpful and important. Satisfaction would have to come from her ability to engage the family in a dialogical praxis that allowed for their greater self-determination. Harder work, no doubt, but without the loss of energy that results from defending against contradictions.

CASE #2: CONTRADICTION RELATED TO RACE AND POWER (POLITICAL JUSTICE)

In part A, Lori, a white student in her late twenties, presented her coleadership of a Curriculum Based Support Group (CBSG) in a southern suburban school with high-risk teens (drug and alcohol use). In each of the twelve planned sessions there was "a check in, an agenda regarding preselected topics/themes thought to affect teen drug use (e.g., anger management, family roles), and some time for open discussion related to the theme."

Lori described her coleader, a white male psychologist, clearly the senior worker to whom she most often deferred, as "a very kind person but a little nervous around tough kids." The school was 90 percent Caucasian, but the thirteen- to eighteen-year-old students in her group were 50 percent Mexican American, 20 percent African American, and 30 percent Caucasian. Though voluntary, students were pressured by the principal and sometimes a probation officer to attend the group.

Lori explained the contradiction she experienced in the following way:

> The kids complained of racist teachers and principal. My coleader and I had some conflict over this. I was told not to rock the boat since the program was very new. I wanted to validate the kids' experience and talk about the racism more but was told not to. . . . The cofacilitator didn't want the kids to get "riled up" with talk of racism. . . . I regrettably followed the direction given.

It needs to be said that Lori did make attempts to engage the group about the topic of racism, which they raised. She asked "if other students or parents complained about racism, if there was a formal way to complain about teachers, and who is a safe person in the school system to talk to about this." But her coleader moved the group away from this discussion and later she was told directly by her supervisor "not to rock the boat." Though she did stop rocking "in order to put her coleader at ease," she "never doubted that what the students described as racism was racism." Students described in other papers for this assignment that they feared jeopardizing their placement if they engaged in social action. We wondered whether Lori also was concerned about this if she persisted in rocking the boat.

In part B, the intervention Lori suggested was to become more active in the group and defer less to her coleader. She believed that if she took a more active role she might be able "to connect the assigned topic with racism and put her coleader at ease." She also imagined that she might be able to get her supervisor to include a session on racism and provide the coleader with a lesson plan she had developed for a teen group she worked with as an undergraduate. She wondered whether becoming more active and engaging the group's outrage, about what they felt was a racially tinged suspension of one of their friends, might have led to social action. Would the group write a letter to the school's administration or get some parents involved? Finally, she believed her friendship with the creator and director of the CBSG project would allow her the access she needed to influence the project.

In part C, Lori explored how the students/clients in her group, her coleader, the director of the CBSG program, and the principal of the school might have reacted to her interventions. She wrote that the "students might have gotten 'riled up' or enthused about the possibility of social action." She recognized, however, that as adolescents they would be concerned about being embarrassed. They would also need to feel that they had truly initiated and planned the social action work. She noted that "the students' ability to request and allow structure and guidance from adults would also bear on the success of the project."

Lori believed her coleader "would be hesitant but would follow whatever direction the director of CBSG provided." The director, whom she knew personally, would be ambivalent. He "would be concerned and talk about racism in the schools" but would also be concerned about his new program and not want to rock the boat. In the end she believed, however hopefully, that he would "suggest a compromise" and allow some small change. Finally, she believed that the principal would be in denial and that any social action "would be used by him as evidence that these kids are 'trouble makers.' "

While recognizing the principal's probable negative reaction, Lori did not seem to fully recognize his power and influence and his ability to squash the project at will. Many students in their papers were either naively optimistic or unduly pessimistic about what was possible. We always encourage positive self-fulfilling prophesies over negative ones. But we also try to temper grandiose fantasies with a bit of reality.

For example, a job and living wage campaign emerged from a staff and resident group one of the authors facilitated at a local homeless shelter. Its goal was to raise the minimum wage to $7.49 an hour. It ultimately took three years to pass a nonbinding resolution before the city council. We do underline that it did pass and that the people who were educated and organized to get it passed can be mobilized for future struggles. We note that social action issues, like intrapsychic issues, take a long time to develop and it takes long-term work and commitment to get real structural change in the mind or in society.

CASE #3: CONTRADICTION RELATED TO DIALOGICAL PRAXIS ACROSS CULTURES

In part A, Abbey, a thirty-year-old white intern, presented the case of Joseph, a thirteen-year-old Haitian-American boy from a single-parent family, who was seen at a short-term inpatient unit of a large teaching hospital. Joseph's symptoms included "unpredictable aggressive behavior, a history of vandalism, nightmares, and hypervigilance." This was Joseph's first hospitalization. His family had a history with the DSS, related to suspected physical abuse by Joseph's mother, Mrs. D, who had immigrated to the United States five years before. In the hospital, Joseph's mother acknowledged hitting him "to make him grow up to be a good boy."

The contradiction for Abbey and the treatment team was related to the obligations they had as mandated reporters. This obligation conflicted with their wish to understand, engage, be respectful of, and dialogue with a family from another culture. The D's were stressed by poverty, immigration, and oppression, and came from a culture that had very different norms about the physical punishment of children. In their attempt to deal with this, the team invited Joseph's mother to be part of the filing with DSS. In addition, the family worker provided information to Mrs. D as follows:

I understand that in Haiti this is the way children are raised, and I understand your worry about feeling like you can't discipline your child without being physical. However, in this country, use of physical punishment like you have used will continue to cause problems with the Department of Social Services. The school and Joseph's therapists must continue to report his bruises to DSS, and they will be investigated. We can try to help you to figure out new ways to deal with discipline in your family if you like, but we have an obligation to let you know that this will continue to be a problem for you in this country if you don't change your discipline style.

Though this information was important and potentially useful, by itself it was limited. As Abbey observed, it sent the message that the problem was between the parent and DSS. The hospital professionals would follow the law, report, and, almost as an afterthought, help her change her behavior. There seemed to be no attempt to dialogue, to ask Mrs. D what she felt and experienced about what was said. There was no attempt to engage her feelings about how she was being treated by DSS or the hospital. Though culture was mentioned, there was no attempt at dialogue between cultures. There was just a short presentation about the consequences for the people of one culture when their behavior did not conform to the laws of the dominant culture. To a worker committed to Freirian practice and dialogical praxis, this is cultural imperialism and a contradiction. Finally, as the instructors suggested in a side comment, the psychological and physical traumas this family likely encountered in Haiti as well as in their migration to the United States would need to be engaged as part of the discussion of the current physical discipline.

In part B, Abbey noted an additional personal/professional contradiction for herself. She believed that clients should come first. In this case she let herself be used as an agent of the state. She reported before any attempts were made to dialogue with the family. Her new intervention would be to discuss the "meaning of discipline versus abuse in both cultures and to reach a mutual plan before or instead of reporting to DSS." Abbey suggested that the issue of discipline and abuse could be problematized, "which would allow for the legal, cultural and personal meanings to be made explicit. . . . [T]he personal violent histories of this son and this mother could be surfaced in a therapeutic way and the alliance could not only be salvaged but strengthened." Finally, in a side note, one of the instructors wondered how this "personal" family issue could be brought to the larger Haitian community of the city, and to what extent was this family's struggle with state law and DSS a social problem that needed to be worked with at a societal level.

In part C, Abbey noted her anxiety as the first consequence of any attempt to implement her intervention. The anxiety had roots both in her inexperience and in the fact that she "would need to look at her own stuff" if she engaged a woman so different from herself who was suspicious of her and rightly saw her as an agent of the larger society.

Other consequences related to her agency, as well as to herself. The agency could get in trouble for not reporting. Because she was a student, if they found out that she was causing trouble they would report her to her supervisor and faculty field advisor. She imagined them first telling her to "knock it off or risk losing her placement." She then asked rhetorically, "Who would be her references when she was looking for a job?" In a side note we answered, "It would be someone who respected what she did and respected her commitment to her values." Finally, Abbey reiterated her commitment to protecting Joseph. "The worst consequence would be if I failed to adequately protect this boy." The question is whether DSS or dialogue will provide the needed protection.

OTHER CASE MATERIAL

Contradictions related to cultural and racial differences and the lack of dialogue were very prevalent in student reports. A white couple hoping to adopt their black foster child neglected, with the agency's acquiescence, to relate to members of the African-American community, including his biological family. Another student felt forced by her supervisor to report to DSS a Puerto Rican mother who curled up in bed with her child. Cultural factors were not taken into account and the family was labeled "enmeshed." Students reported that agencies serving African-American clients showed little inclination, in spite of values to the contrary, to hire African-American staff. Agency staff and students often found that it was more expedient to do something for a new immigrant than to work through the language difficulties that would allow the client more self-determination.

Staff and students who valued therapeutic dialogue would give in to senior staff, and particularly senior clinicians, who were actively abusive and punitive toward clients. One doctor, in what sounded like malpractice, required "total submission from patients or he would remove medication." He suggested parents lock their children in their rooms for hours at a time until they "learned their lesson." In fear of reprisals or loss of jobs, staff kept silent and students were encouraged to do the same.

An increasingly recurrent theme in the papers was that clients who needed long-term work were given short-term care. The profit needs of managed care insurers have clearly compromised the value of client-focused treatment.

Students also wrote about the real limitations some clients had in effecting change. For example, a student worked with an undocumented immigrant family. She was well aware of and understood their limits in going public with their difficulties related to immigration. She knew she would need to work apart from this family to change oppressive immigration laws that affected them. Nevertheless, she noted how dialogue with this family could strengthen family relationships and build trust with the worker.

Other students posed more pessimistic consequences. White staff would be uptight if an African American was hired for a position of power. Staff who were put on the spot or asked to change might scapegoat clients. Supervisors would be anxious about their own status in the agency and not be supportive. Faculty field advisors and the School would be concerned about preserving a "good" placement. Students would be told to "cool it."

ADDITIONAL COMMENTS

In the review of the papers, a number of general themes and issues emerged. Considering them will be useful to students and faculty attempting to do the work discussed in this book.

The concept of contradiction was often discussed in an imprecise way. For that reason, it was extremely important to revisit this central concept in the discussion of the written assignment and again when we returned part A of the paper. As we noted in Chapter 7, students need to be clear about the difference between a contradiction and other kinds of conflicts or issues. For this reason, we ask them to provide specific examples of what they describe in their papers as contradictions. We want to know what value that is being contradicted and how their behavior or the agency's practices places them in a contradiction with that value.

A related issue is that students often report on two values which are in conflict and the inevitable contradiction that occurs. They are often unclear about the actual meaning and implications of their personal and professional values. Even when they are clear, students have not yet arrived at a consistent ordering of those values. This is difficult as there is constant change in the contexts within which the values they hold are tested.

In part B, as we ask students to look at alternative interventions, other issues emerge. A common one is that, in their wish to do social action, they assume a heroic stance that entails doing for the client rather than dialoguing with clients. This is in contradiction to the values of self-determination and dialogical praxis. At this stage of their praxis, it is unclear whether their interventions are grounded in a conflict with the values we put forward or merely in a lack of skill.

Related to these issues is the students' anxiety about trying something new. They recognize their limitations and have concerns about their competence. Are they actually able to dialogue with clients? If they did, could they then bring the substance of the dialogue to their agencies for action? They were anxious about getting into trouble at their agencies.

In part C, students had difficulty recognizing, tolerating, and appreciating the process of change. On one hand, they did not acknowledge real resistances to change in individuals and institutions. They were sometimes unwilling or unable to recognize their own limitations and those of their clients. They did not appreciate the painfully slow pace of organizational change. On the other hand, some were willing to concede defeat too quickly and imagined themselves as absolutely powerless in the face of overwhelming odds.

Our approach to responding to the students' papers was to view this as an opportunity for dialogue. In this spirit, we attempt to help clarify issues, raise questions, and suggest readings and strategies, such as documenting incidents.

We are encouraging about their willingness to reflect authentically on their work and the risks they contemplate taking. We note how agencies sometimes act in ways that recapitulate a client's trauma, such as abandoning children who have been abandoned or not listening to people who never received attention. We make some attempts at humor. Finally, we talk about the need to rest and take care of oneself, "to get by with a little help from our friends."

We end here with a quote from James Baldwin that one of our students used to end her paper. "Not everything that is faced can be changed. But nothing can be changed until it is faced."

Epilogue

Both of the authors came into the field in the 1960s when the false dichotomy was skewed toward social action. In the years since, as the political climate has become more conservative, the skew in the dichotomy has shifted back to clinical work. And the clinical work itself has been narrowed by the forces of managed care. The ascendancy of managed care has its roots in the emergence and growth of private practice in the 1970s and 1980s. Social workers have become small business owners, capitalists. More than half of social workers, according to NASW, are engaged in some form of private practice. We believe that managed care insurance companies are the logical outcome of the move toward privatization and private practice, in a capitalist society run amok. Big companies take over small ones, chickens come home to roost.

In this climate, it is increasingly difficult to practice from the values outlined in this book. These values, we believe, are at their core both radical and optimistic. Though we became social workers in the 1960s, we remember the 1950s when the forces of conservatism had a stranglehold on the country and it was dangerous to voice and act on progressive ideas. Times changed and, we believe, they will again. For them to change, a vision of hope must be kept alive. In the spirit of Paulo Freire, we try to advance a "pedagogy of hope" in our class and, we hope, throughout this book.

A consistent theme in the years we have taught this class has been that students ask us how we maintain both hope and energy. These questions have forced us to reflect and we have, over the years, come to a greater clarity of what is needed to keep a vision alive in times that do not sustain it. What we have said to them, and we would like to say to you, is the following.

We believe that, to do this work, people need to have a source of transcendent values which fuels them and to which they can return. For us, this source is our heritage as Jews, a tradition that has an ethical base, is grounded in critical thought, and has a tragic history that sensitizes us to injustice. One of the authors grew up during the Holocaust; the other's experience was shaped by the history of his parents' escape from Hitler's Germany.

Both authors are members of the Bertha Capen Reynolds Society, a national organization of progressive workers in social welfare. Our affiliation provides relationships with people who share our ideas, our commitments, and our need to play.

The work we describe takes place over a long period of time, over generations. The intensity that this demands must be tempered with rest, self-care, and nurturing relationships. Another way to describe this is that we need balance in our lives. Family and loving relationships are a necessary counterweight to the harsh realities that provoke our outrage. Taking time out to experience beauty is an antidote to the ugliness in the world.

Finally, we have no choice. The alternative, doing nothing, is unacceptable. We end with the words of the courageous Russian poet, Yevtushenko (1962), who concluded his poem "Lies" with this warning to parents and teachers who do not tell the young of the difficulties and hardships

and afterwards our [children and] pupils
will not forgive in us what we forgave.

Appendix A

Process Recording—Mary, 10/11/90

Mary arrived ten minutes late for the session. J is a student worker.

M: I thought it would take me only ten minutes to get here, but it took more like twenty. I'm sorry I'm late.

J: Well, OK. You'll know next time how long it takes you to get here.

M: Yeah. [A little breathless.]

J: It's been two weeks since we've seen each other, Mary. How are you?

M: Wow, what a question. How am I? Yes, it's been a pretty hectic two weeks, too, with everything that's happened, especially in the past few days.

J: Well, I guess I've got some catching up to do. What's been going on?

M: Let's see. Where to begin? I'm really concerned about my boyfriend. I don't know where to start. I guess I'm mostly concerned about the fact that he's gotten a hold of a handgun and, well, he's been acting pretty strange lately.

J: So, you're concerned about what he might want to do with a handgun?

M: Yeah. It was weird. Things have not been going well for him.

(Mary proceeds to tell how her boyfriend has lost his job and as a result will have to quit school because work was subsidizing his coursework. Although Mary has been distancing from this boyfriend for the past two months, and they have had fights, she felt sorry for him and went to his apartment to console him on Saturday.)

M: He was talking pretty crazy and I was just trying to, you know, say nice things to him, try to calm him down. It seemed like the longer I stayed, though, the weirder he got. He had this gun out and he'd been cleaning it while we were talking. I started to feel weird about being there the more we talked. So, I made some excuse, but I said, "I'm sorry about what you're going through, Larry." And I started to leave. He stood up then, and pointed the gun right at me. He said, "Yeah, you're gonna leave me, Mary?" Real crazy. He was calling me names and just losing it. I didn't know what to do or what to say, so I just backed out of there and ran away. I ran and ran, I left my car behind I was so scared. I ran to a friend's house and told him what had happened, and gave him my keys and he went back and got my car for me. He said that when he went he could see Larry sitting on the porch in front of the door, just holding the gun and staring. My friend didn't know if Larry saw him or not, but he didn't say or do anything.

J: Sounds like you were very frightened, Mary.

M: I really was. I thought about it afterward and I don't know if maybe I overreacted.

J: You think you may have overreacted?

M: Well, I think he was in a really crazy frame of mind, but I don't think he would have shot me.

J: Maybe not, Mary. But I think you were in danger. Although you know Larry as someone who cares about you and has cared for you, you were in danger.

M: Yeah, I guess even if he didn't mean to pull the trigger, the gun could have gone off. He even took the safety off.

J: It sounds like you did exactly what you needed to do to take care of yourself and exactly what your instincts told you to do.

M: Right. I wasn't thinking. I just ran.

J: Have you contacted the police?

M: Yes, I did. I called and talked for some time to a detective. He was very helpful.

(Mary described her conversation with the detective. She and the detective apparently went through all of Mary's options very thoroughly, including predicting what would be likely to happen if Mary pressed charges for assault, which she was in a position to do, if she chose. The upshot of the conversation was that it wasn't illegal for Larry to own a gun and that it was unlikely that pressing charges would result in the gun being confiscated from him. The officer also felt it was unlikely that Larry would be held for very long if he were arrested. Mary felt that in the long run it would do her very little good to see the thing through and might put her in further danger but felt guilty for not taking legal action.)

J: What's the guilt about, Mary?

M: If I don't do something about this, will Larry hurt himself? Or somebody else? At this point he probably won't do anything to hurt me, or at least now I don't think so. I wasn't so sure last night.

J: What do you mean?

M: Well, I think he might have camped out behind my apartment building last night. I saw a campfire and beer cans and the dog was making funny noises and wagging his tail when we went for a walk. Like he recognized someone. It's how he acts when he sees Larry.

J: You thought Larry might have been there?

M: I did.

J: What did you do?

M: Well, it was lucky. My father was over for dinner and I asked him to stay. I told him I was nervous because Larry's been weird lately. He stayed till midnight and nothing happened after that. But I didn't get much sleep last night.

J: You were pretty nervous.

M: Yeah. I guess I could have gone back there, just to see. But I was so scared. And it's crazy because maybe he was there, but maybe not.

J: You don't know for sure. But it's clear that this has you feeling pretty terrorized.

M: God, yes.

J: Having someone point a loaded gun at you is a traumatizing thing. It wouldn't surprise me if you felt frightened and jumpy in the aftermath. Let's talk about some things you can do to manage it when you feel afraid.

(Solutions were explored for times when Mary felt afraid because she was alone, or suspected she was in danger. Alerting her father to the situation was the first possibility discussed. Mary was reluctant to tell her father about what had happened when she went to Larry's because he had been against her relationship with him from the beginning.)

M: It will upset him. Really it will just open up a can of worms and I don't think I'll end up with much more support.

J: What does your father know about your relationship with Larry?

M: Well, he knows I'm still seeing him, but that we've had some rough times. He knows things are bad right now. I told him that when he was over for dinner, but he'd flip if I told him about the gun and everything.

J: He'd be . . .

M: He'd be concerned, but . . .

J: Is it an "I told you so" experience you'd like to avoid?

M: Yes. I don't need to hear that from him right now.

J: Mary, is there anything you can tell your father that would get you a little more support from him right now? I mean, something honest, but that won't get you into the "I told you so" discussion?

M: Well, I guess I could tell him how scared I feel. ·

J: That might be a good approach. He knows Larry's been acting strangely now?

M: Yes, he does.

J: So if you told him you might need him to check up on you a little more frequently, or to be around a bit more in the next few days . . .

M: He would do that. Absolutely. He's always come through for me, OK.

(The next possibility I suggested was for Mary to pay attention to her feelings, particularly those that indicated she was not safe, and to take action. She should listen to her gut.)

M: You mean, if I think Larry is outside the house again?

J: Exactly.

M: Hmmm. What could I do?

J: Can you think of anything?

M: Besides locking the doors?

J: That's good. Anything else? [pause] How about calling the police and having them send a cruiser to check out the premises?

M: Really?

J: Really. What do you think of that?

M: Well, I guess I might do that, but I'd feel strange. I mean you feel so silly.

J: It might be a false alarm? How convinced are you that Larry was outside your house?

M: I *know* he was there. But what if they don't come?

J: You might call them in advance and find out if they would come if you called. Let them know the situation.

M: Yeah. I could do that. I already called to ask about a restraining order. They said it wasn't really a possibility since he lives in Maryland.

J: Really. That sounds strange.

M: I thought so too.

(The last possible action we looked at was to contact neighbors and let them know Larry was not welcome at Mary's house and to ask them to keep an eye out. Mary had already done this and her close friends knew of the situation. She felt comfortable calling on any of them when she felt frightened.)

J: Mary, I'd like to go back to when you said you were feeling guilty.

M: Yeah. I know I shouldn't feel guilt or responsibility for Larry or really for anyone but myself. I know that intellectually.

J: But you're not totally convinced.

M: No. But this is typical for me. Real typical of how I am in relationships. I know I do this. I do anything to keep other people from getting angry. If I hurt anyone or make them mad, I feel so guilty. And I'm afraid for Larry right now. I know I'm not responsible for his well-being, but, well, I've acted that way so long with him, I don't really know how to stop.

J: What might happen if you were to stop feeling responsible for Larry?

M: When we were together, he might leave me. That sounds crazy, because I didn't even know if I wanted to be with him. He was so mean to me, said so many terrible things to me. I hurt from that. But I still am afraid of being alone.

J: How do you feel about the relationship with Larry right now?

M: I don't know. If he were to come to me and apologize for what he did and beg me to take him back. I'd like to say I won't. But I can't be sure. You know I talked to someone about the support groups at CASA. They sound like they're really good and the more I hear about women who get abused, the more I think I'm like that.

J: You've done some investigating into this?

M: I've done some reading.

J: And you saw some of yourself in that.

M: Not that I've been physically abused. But it's like abuse, when someone constantly criticizes and makes you feel like shit about yourself. And that was true in other relationships too. James' father [the father of her son] was like that. One minute I was great and the next I was awful, not worth a moment of his time.

J: If you're interested, Mary, I think it might be very worthwhile for you to call CASA and ask about joining a support group. That's the kind of work that is real appropriate to do while you're in individual therapy too.

M: I wondered about that. It's OK to do both?

J: Absolutely. If you found the group worthwhile, I would support your continuing with it.

M: OK. I'll call them.

J: We have just about ten minutes left, Mary, and what we're talking about reminds me of the fact that this is your third session and our original contract was to use three sessions to explore what it was you'd like to work on in therapy and set some goals.

M: Oh, yeah. Well, this is certainly one of them, I think.

J: I remember when you first came in you mentioned some patterns you saw in your relationships . . .

M: Yeah, this is what I was talking about. I'd like to work on this stuff. It seems like I have some sick need that keeps on cropping up. I have no idea where it comes from or what it's about. But whatever it is, it keeps me in bad relationships. It makes me not very much fun to be with sometimes. I guess my self-esteem must be pretty low or something for me to want to be in such lousy relationships.

J: You have needs that seem unhealthy to you right now.

M: Yeah, because they're so all-encompassing, I just lose it when I think I'm going to be alone. I end up doing things I regret.

J: Your needs are so all-encompassing that they seem unhealthy. Sometimes the need to be loved and cared for seems large and out of proportion because it's been unmet for a long time. Beginning with parents, if they were unable to meet your needs because they were caught up in their own problems.

M: Yeah,

J: Maybe we could say that your need to be loved is very great, very big.

M: Huge.

J: But fundamentally, it is a healthy need, Mary [pause]. Have you thought much about what it is you'd like to get in a relationship?

M: Not that much.

J: How about the ways you'd like your needs to be met in a relationship?

M: I've mostly thought about what I don't want.

J: That's important to know too. We're out of time, but I'd like to propose a bit of homework for us to talk about for next time.

M: OK.

J: Pretend that you're about to begin your ideal relationship. What would you look forward to about the relationship? What would it be like? What needs would be met in a healthy way? You can write down your thoughts about this if you like.

M: I don't know if I can do it.

J: What would keep you from being able to?

M: I don't know what I want.

J: OK. Another way to think about this might be to try to pinpoint the things about your past relationships that *have* been good for you. Could you try that?

M: I could.

J: There's no failing with this, Mary. If it doesn't seem helpful to try this during the week, we can look at it together next week, OK?

M: OK.

J: OK. We need to stop now. Let's talk more about this next week.

Appendix B

Process Recording—
Ben Williams and Frank, 1/27/98

Notes: Ninth session
C = Client (Frank)
W = Worker (Ben)

C: Hello, Mr. Williams.
W: Hello, Frank.
C: Did you get the money order I sent?
W: Yeah, I got the money order.
C: I got some money for today and I can pay the rest that I owe when I get paid next week.
W: That's good, Frank, I'm glad to see you're being more responsible . . . how does it feel to be working and able to do more for yourself financially?
C: It feels good . . . I mean I feel like I'm getting myself together.
W: Is there a difference between how you feel about yourself now as opposed to before when you were not doing so well?
C: Yeah . . . [pause] . . . it's like . . . before I really didn't care about too much . . . I didn't feel good about myself . . . [long pause] . . . now I think more about things . . . I feel better about myself.
W: I'm happy to see you're feeling better about yourself now . . . I'm wondering though . . . What do you think is the reason for your doing better now? What has changed?
C: Lisa . . . she helped me a lot . . . I mean since I been with her I've calmed down a lot. I'm more settled down now. Plus, I'm getting older now. I'm not getting no younger.
W: I see . . . but what do you think has changed within you to make you look at things the way you do now?
C: [long pause] I don't know . . . I guess I gotta think about that . . . [long pause] I mean I got a baby on the way, she's due in June. I wasn't

209

really there for the rest of my kids so I want to be there for this one . . . I got to change for this kid . . . I want my kid to respect me.

W: It sounds like this new baby has motivated you a lot to change.

C: Yeah, but not just the baby . . . Lisa too . . . I want us to get along better.

W: So how are you getting along?

C: We're doing OK. . . . We're actually talking about getting married.

W: Isn't she still legally married?

C: Yeah, but she's filing the papers now . . . we're thinking about going to Las Vegas in the summer and getting married.

W: How do you feel about getting married?

C: I'm happy about it . . . I know we got some problems to work out but I think we can do it.

W: How does Lisa feel about it?

C: She wants it too . . . she's happy about it.

W: Now, I notice you look a little tired.

C: Yeah, I been working a lot lately.

W: So how is the job going?

C: It's going good, they got me working the movie projector now . . . it's OK. . . . [pause] . . . Oh, yeah, did you hear about what happened the other day at the movie theater?

W: No, tell me what happened.

C: This kid got stabbed for his coat . . . he died too.

W: Were you there when this happened?

C: Yeah, but I didn't see it . . . I was working the projector . . . the kid was only about eighteen or nineteen years old . . . it was sad.

W: Who stabbed him?

C: I don't know who the guy was but he wanted his coat and the kid told him he can have it but he stabbed the kid anyway. It kinda shook me up . . . It made me cry . . . I been a little disturbed about it lately.

W: Why do you think it made you feel that way?

C: 'Cause I don't understand it . . . I mean I thought people had stopped doing stuff like that.

W: So it sounds like you were able to feel a sense of loss.

C: Yeha, . . . it was a life cut short. It don't make no sense . . . not to kill someone over a coat. I wish I could see the guy who did it.

W: What would you say or do to him?

C: I would tell him he's stupid . . . stupid . . . messing up his whole life for a coat . . . hurting himself, his family. Also the family of the kid who died, they're going through a lot now . . . they're hurting. I heard the kid was a good guy too . . . he was going to college, he didn't get into any trouble . . . [long pause] . . . I met the kid's father too . . . his father came to the theater to see where it happened and where his son was sitting. My supervisor had me escort him . . . I was real nervous. I didn't even know what to say to him.

W: Did you say anything to him?

C: Yeah, I told him I was sorry about what happened to his son . . . he was real shaken up, he asked me why someone would do something like this . . . I told him I don't know. He and his family set up a memorial at the theater. I seen them come to set it up. They were all crying . . . that was hard to see.

W: So it sounds like this was pretty traumatic for you.

C: Yeah, . . . [long pause] . . . I felt really bad for the family . . . Yeah and the cops came to the theater to talk to all of us . . . I didn't really feel comfortable talking to them.

W: Why? How did it feel for you?

C: I guess it felt like I was in trouble . . . it reminded me of times when I got arrested before. I felt like I was locked up again.

W: So do you think about your past troubles a lot?

C: Sometimes . . . but usually when something like this happens.

W: Does thinking about your past affect the way you feel about what happened?

C: Yeah . . . I think that it could have been me . . . either killing somebody or getting killed myself . . . [long pause] . . . before, I didn't care about nothing. I didn't really care if I lived or died.

W: And how do you feel now?

C: Now I do care . . . about myself . . . Lisa, my family.

W: So you feel like you have something to live for, a reason to get your life together?

C: Yeah, now I do.

W: So do you have any feelings or thoughts about what happened?

C: [pause] I guess it scared me a little.

W: Tell me what scared you.

C: Well, I think something like that could happen to me . . . these young 'uns today act like I did when I was younger . . . and they still ain't caught the guy who stabbed him yet. He still on the run. . . . I could run into this guy one day.

W: It sounds like this tragedy had made you think a lot about your past and also triggered some fears for you.

C: Yeah . . . [long pause]

W: What are some of your fears?

C: [long pause] I guess I think that my past might catch up to me someday . . . or now that I'm trying to get myself together something will happen.

W: How often do you think about these fears?

C: Not that often, usually when something like this happens.

W: Well, I think it's natural to feel that way sometimes . . . before you didn't really care about anything. When you don't care about anything and nothing has any value, including yourself, there is nothing really to fear. When you care about yourself and others it's only natural to worry sometimes. We all have fears when we care about something.

C: Yeah . . . I think I see what you saying. It's like before I had nothing to lose so I wasn't afraid of anything. Now I feel like I got something to lose so I get afraid sometimes.

W: That's right, that's a good way of looking at it . . . It sounds like you are able to see the difference between how you looked at things then as opposed to now.

C: Yeah . . . [long pause] Now if I didn't change the way I was, I was only gonna end up back in jail or worse . . . now I try to talk to the young 'uns at work . . . they be talking about stealing cars, selling drugs. I be telling them stories about things I did and what happened to me. I tell them I know it's all fun now but it's not worth it in the long run.

W: So how does it feel to talk to younger guys about some of the things you've done in the past?

C: It's OK. I don't feel as bad about it now that I'm doing better.

W: I see we're about out of time but I wanted to see if there was anything else you wanted to talk about today.

C: No, not really. . . . but I did want to talk to you about some of the stuff I've been reading.

W: That's fine, why don't you bring some of the stuff you've been reading in next week and we can go over it.

C: OK, I'll do that.

Bibliography

Abramovitz, M. (1988). *Regulating the lives of women.* Boston: South End Press.

Abramovitz, M. (1996). *Under attack, fighting back: Women and welfare in the United States.* New York: Monthly Review Press.

Alexander, C. A. (1991). Creating and using coalitions. In R. L. Edwards and J. A. Yankey (Eds.), *Skills for effective human service management.* Washington. DC: NASW Press, pp. 90-102.

Amidei, N. (1982). How to be an advocate in bad times. *Public Welfare,* Summer, 37-42.

Aronowitz, S. (1993). Paulo Freire's radical democratic humanism. In P. McLaren and P. Leonard (Eds.), *Paulo Freire: A critical encounter.* London and New York: Routledge, pp. 8-24.

Baekeland, F. and Lundwall, L. (1975). Dropping out of treatment: A critical review. *Psychological Bulletin, 82(5):* 738-783.

Bailey, R. and Brake, M. (1975). *Radical social work.* New York: Pantheon.

Bartlett, H. (1970). *The common base of social work practice.* Washington, DC: National Association of Social Workers.

Bateson, G. (1979). *Mind and nature.* New York: E. P. Dutton.

Berger, P. I. (1963). *Invitation to sociology.* Garden City, NY: Anchor Books.

Berger, P. and Luckmann, T. (1966). *The social construction of reality.* New York: Anchor Books.

Bernstein, N. (1997). Deletion of one word in welfare bill opens foster care to big business. *The New York Times,* May 4, pp. 1, 26.

Blackwell, J. E. and Janowitz, M. (1974). *Black sociologists: Historical and contemporary perspectives.* Chicago: The University of Chicago Press.

Blau, J. (1992). *The visible poor.* New York: Oxford University Press.

Bloch, E. (1966). Man and citizen according to Marx. In E. Fromm (Ed.), *Socialist humanism.* Garden City, NY: Anchor Books, pp. 220-227.

Bobo, K., Kendall, J., and Max, S. (1991). *Organizing for social change: A manual for activists in the 1990's.* Washington, DC: Seven Locks Press.

Bock, S. (1980). Conscientization: Paulo Freire and class-based practice. *Catalyst,* 6, 5-25.

Boyd-Franklin, N. (1989). *Black families in therapy.* New York: Guilford Press.

Brager, G. and Holloway, S. (1978). *Changing human services organizations: Politics and practice.* New York: Free Press.

Bramson, L. (1961). *The political context of sociology.* Princeton, NJ: Princeton University Press.

Briar, K. and Briar, S. (1981). Clinical social work and public policies. In M. Mahaffey and J. Hanks (Eds.), *Practical politics: Social workers and political action.* Silver Spring, MD: NASW, pp. 45-54.

Bricker-Jenkins, M. and Hooyman, N. (1986). *Not for women only.* Silver Spring, MD: NASW.

Burghardt, S. (1982). *The other side of organizing.* Rochester, VT: Schenkman Books.

Burstow, B. (1991). Freirian codifications and social work education. *Journal of Social Work Education, 27*(2), 196-207.

Camus, A. (1955). *The myth of Sisyphus.* New York: Vintage.

Carlson, B. E. (1977). Battered women and their assailants. *Social Work, 22* (November), 455-460.

Cerbone, A. R. (1991). The effects of political activism on psychotherapy: A case study. In C. Silverstein (Ed.), *Gays, lesbians, and their therapists.* New York: W. W. Norton and Company, pp. 40-51.

Cloward, R. A. and Piven., F. F. (1976), Note toward a radical social work. In F. Bailey and M. Brake (Eds.), *Radical social work.* New York: Pantheon, pp. vii-xlviii.

Collins, P. H. (1991). *Black feminist thought.* New York: Routledge.

Connerton, P. (1976). *Critical sociology.* Harmondsworth, England: Penguin.

Cooley, C. H. (1964). The primacy of primary groups. In *Mass society in crisis.* Rosenberg, B., I. Gerver, and W. F. Howton. (Eds.), New York: Macmillan Company, 70-74.

Cooper, S. (1977). Social work: A dissenting profession. *Social Work, 22*(5), 360-368.

Coser, L. A. and Rosenberg, B. (1969). *Sociological theory: A book of readings,* Third edition. New York: The Macmillan Co.

Davis, A. Y. (1983). *Women, race and class.* New York: Vintage.

Davis, L. V. (1987). Battered women: The transformation of a social problem. *Social Work, 32* (July-August), 306-311.

Dear, R. and Patti, R. (1982). Legislative advocacy: Seven effective tactics. In M. Mahaffey and J. Hanks (Eds.), *Practical politics: Social workers and political action.* Silver Spring, MD: NASW, pp. 99-117.

Debs, E. V. (1966). A sentiment on social reform. As cited in U. Sinclair (Ed.), *The cry for justice: An anthology of the great social protest literature of all time.* New York: Barricade Books, p. 110.

DeMonteflores, C. (1981). Conflicting allegiances: Therapy issues with Hispanic lesbians. *Catalyst, 12,* 31-36.

DeMott, B. (1996). Seduced by civility: Political manners and the crisis of democratic values. *The Nation,* December 9, 11-19.

Dolgoff, R. and Gordon, M. (1981). Education for policy-making at the direct service and local level. *Journal of Social Work Education, 17*(2), 98-105.

Dujon, D. and Withorn, A. (1996). *For crying out loud: Women's poverty in the United States.* Boston: South End Press.

Ehrenreich, J. and Ehrenreich, B. (1979). The professional managerial class. In P. Walker (Ed.), *Between labor and capital.* Boston: South End Press, pp. 5-45.

Eissler, K. (1953). The effect of the structure of the ego on psychoanalytic technique. *Journal of the American Psychoanalytic Association, 1*(1), 104-143.

Etzioni, A. (1969). *The semi-professions and their organizations.* New York: Free Press.

Fabricant, M. and Burghardt, S. (1992). *The welfare state crisis and the transformation of social service work.* Armonk, NY: M. E. Sharpe, Inc.

Fanon, F. (1967). *Black skins, white masks.* New York: Grove Press.

Findlay, P. C. (1978). Critical theory and social work practice. *Catalyst, 3,* 53-68.

Fisher, R. (1984). *Let the people decide.* Boston: Twayne.

Flanagan, J. C. (1954). The critical incident technique. *Psychological Bulletin, 51*(4), 327-358.

Freire, P. (1985). *The politics of education.* South Hadley, MA: Bergin and Garvey.

Freire, P. (1989a). *Pedagogy of the oppressed.* New York: Continuum. Reprinted by permission of the Continuum Publishing Company.

Freire, P. (1989b). *Education for critical consciousness.* New York: Continuum.

Freire, P. (1990). A critical understanding of social work. *Journal of Progressive Human Services, 1*(1), 3-9.

Freire, P. (1998). *Teachers as cultural workers: Letters to those who dare teach.* Boulder, CO: Westview Press.

Freire, P. and Macedo, D. (1987). *Literacy: Reading the word and the world.* South Hadley, MA: Bergin and Garvey.

Freud, A. (1966). *The ego and the mechanisms of defense.* New York: International Universities Press.

Freud, S. (1900). *The interpretation of dreams, standard edition* (J. Strachey, Trans.). London: Hogarth Press.

Freud, S. (1949). *An outline of psycho-analysis.* New York: W. W. Norton and Company. (Original work published 1940.)

Freud, S. (1955). *Studies in hysteria.* New York: Basic Books. (Original work published 1893.)

Freud, S. (1959). *Inhibitions, symptoms and anxiety.* (A. Strachey, Trans.) New York: W. W. Norton and Co. (Original work published 1926.)

Freud, S. (1962a). *Civilization and its discontents* (J. Strachey, Trans.). New York: W.W. Norton and Co. (Original work published 1930.)

Freud, S. (1962b). *Three essays on the theory of sexuality* (J. Strachey, Trans.). New York: Basic Books. (Original work published 1905.)

Freud, S. (1963a). Analysis terminable and interminable. In P. Reiff (Ed.), *Therapy and technique.* New York: Collier Books. (Original work published 1937.)

Freud, S. (1963b). The dynamics of transference. In P. Reiff (Ed.), *Therapy and technique,* New York: Collier Books. (Original work published 1912.)

Freud, S. (1963c). Instincts and their vicissitudes. In *General psychological theory.* New York: Collier Books. (Original work published 1915.)

Freud, S. (1963d). Negation. In *General psychological theory.* New York: Collier Books. (Original work published 1925.)

Freud, S. (1963e). Remembering, repeating and working through. In P Reiff (Ed.), *Therapy and technique.* New York: Collier Books. (Original work published 1914.)

Freud, S. (1963f). The unconscious. In *General psychological theory.* New York: Collier Books. (Original work published 1915.)

Freud, S. (1964). *New introductory lectures on psychoanalysis* (J. Strachey, Trans.). New York: W.W. Norton and Co. (Original work published 1933.)

Freud, S. (1965). *New introductory lectures on psychoanalysis.* (J. Strachey, Trans.) New York: W. W. Norton and Co. (Original work published 1932.)

Freund, J. (1969). *The sociology of Max Weber.* New York: Vintage.

Fromm, E. (1966). The application of humanist psychoanalysis to Marx's theory. In E. Fromm (Ed.), *Socialist humanism.* Garden City, NY: Anchor Books, pp. 228-245.

Fromm, E. (1972). Karl Marx's theory of alienation. In D. Wrong and H. Gracey, (Eds.), *Readings in introductory sociology,* Second edition. New York: Macmillan, pp. 188-195. (Original work published 1961.)

Galper, J. (1973). Personal politics and psychoanalysis. *Social Policy, 4*(3), 35-43.

Galper, J. (1978). Social welfare in capitalist society: A socialist analysis. *Catalyst, 1.*

Garfinkel, H. (1956). Conditions of successful degradation ceremonies. In L. Hazelrigg (Ed.) (1968), *Prison within society.* Garden City, NY: Anchor Books, pp. 68-77.

Garfinkel, H. (1967). *Studies in ethnomethodology.* Englewood Cliffs, NJ: Prentice-Hall.

Germain, C. B. and Gitterman, A. (1980). *The life model of social work practice.* New York: Columbia University Press.

Gil, D. (1978). Clinical practice and the politics of human liberation. *Catalyst, 2,* 61-69.

Gilbert, N. and Specht, H. (1976). Advocacy and professional ethics. *Social Work, 21* (July), 288-293.

Gilder, G. (1981). *Wealth and poverty.* New York: Bantam Books.

Gill, M. (1980). The analysis of the transference. In H. P. Blum (Ed.), *Psychoanalytic explorations of technique.* New York: International Universities Press, pp. 263-288.

Gilman, S. L. (1993). *Freud, race and gender.* Princeton, NJ: Princeton University Press.

Glaser, B. G. and Strauss, A. L. (1967). *The discovery of grounded theory.* Chicago: Aldine.

Goffman, E. (1961). *Asylums.* Garden City, NY: Anchor Books.

Goffman, E. (1963). *Stigma.* Englewood Cliffs, NJ: Prentice-Hall.

Gorden, W. and Schutz, M. L. (1977). A natural base for social work specializations. *Social Work, 22* (September), 422-426.

Gordon, W. (1962). A critique of the working definition. *Social Work, 7.*

Gouldner, A. W. (1970). *The coming crisis of western sociology.* New York: Equinox.

Greenson, R. (1967). *The technique and practice of psychoanalysis.* New York: International Universities Press.

Groddeck, G. (1977). *The meaning of illness.* New York: International Universities Press.

Guralnik, D. B. (Ed.). (1970). *Webster's new world dictionary of the American language: Second college edition.* New York: The World Publishing Company.

Hartman, H. (1958). *Ego psychology and the problems of adaptation.* New York: International Universities Press.

Hasenfeld, Y. (1987). Power in social work practice. *Social Service Review, 61*(3), 469-480.

Haynes, K. and Mickelson, J. (1986). *Affecting change: Social workers in the political arena.* New York: Longman.

Heaney, T. (1997). Issues in Freirian pedagoogy. <http://nlu.nl.edu/ace/Resources/Documents/FreireIssues.html>.

Herrnstein, R. and Murray, C. (1994). *The bell curve: Intelligence and class structure in American life.* New York: Free Press.

Hofstadter, R. (1955). *Social Darwinism in American thought.* Boston: Beacon Press.

hooks, b. (1994). *Teaching to transgress.* New York: Rutledge.

Horkheimer, M. (1937). Traditional and critical theory. In P. Connerton (Ed.), (1976), *Critical sociology.* Harmondsworth, England: Penguin, pp. 206-224. (Original work published 1937.)

Horton, M. and Freire, P. (1990). *We make the road by walking.* Philadelphia: Temple University Press.

Husserl, E. (1967). *The Paris lectures* (P. Koestenbaum, Trans.). The Hague: Martinus Nijhoff.

James, C. E. (1995). *Perspectives on racism and the human services sector.* Toronto: University of Toronto Press.

Jeffrey, N. A. (1988). A new balancing act for psychiatry. *The Wall Street Journal,* January 5, B1, B7.

Jorden, J. (1985). *On call.* Boston: South End Press.

Kahn, S. (1991). *Organizing.* Washington: NASW Press.

Kearney, L. (1970). Anxiety. In H. Nagera (Ed.), *Basic psychoanalytic concepts: On metapsychology, conflicts, anxiety and other subjects.* London: Maresfield Reprints, pp. 127-129.

Kinoy, S. (1984). Advocacy: A potent antidote to burnout. *NASW News,* November, 9.

Langs, R. (1981). *Classics in psycho-analytic technique.* New York: Jason Aronson.

Lee, J. (1994). *The empowerment approach to social work practice.* New York: Columbia University Press.

Lefkowitz, R. and Withorn, A. (1986). *For crying out loud.* New York: The Pilgrim Press.

Leonard, P. (1975). Toward a paradigm for radical practice. In R. Bailey and M. Brake (Eds.), *Radical social work.* New York: Pantheon, pp. 46-61.

Leonard, P. (1993). Critical pedagogy and state welfare: Intellectual encounters with Freire and Gramsci, 1974-88. In P. McLaren and P. Leonard (Eds.), *Paulo Freire: A critical encounter.* London and New York: Routledge, pp. 155-168.

Leonard, S. T. (1990). *Critical theory in political practice.* Princeton, NJ: Princeton University Press.

Lieberman, A. (1988). Internal representations of community. Unpublished master's thesis, Smith College School for Social Work, Northampton, MA.

Little, M. (1981). Counter-transference and the patient's response to it. In R. Langs (Ed.), *Classics in psycho-analytic technique.* New York: Jason Aronson, pp. 143-152. (Original work published 1951.)

Litwak, E. (1960). Occupational mobility and family cohesion. *American Sociological Review, 25*(1), 9-21.

Lowenberg, F. and Dolgoff, R. (1982) *Ethical decisions for social work practice.* Itasca, IL: Peacock.

Lubove, R. (1972). *The professional altruist.* New York: Atheneum.

Luckmann, T. (1978). *Phenomenology and sociology.* New York: Penguin.

Lundblad, K. S. (1995). Jane Addams and social reform: A role model for the 1990s. *Social Work, 40* (September), 661-669.

Maglin, A. (1978). Social values and psychotherapy. *Catalyst, 3,* 69-79.

Manis, J. G. and Meltzer, B. N. (1967). *Symbolic interaction: A reader in social psychology,* Second edition. Boston: Allyn and Bacon.

Marcuse, H. (1962). *Eros and civilization.* New York: Vintage.

Marcuse, H. (1966). *One-dimensional man.* Boston: Beacon Press.

Marcuse, H. (1969). *An essay on liberation.* Boston: Beacon Press.

Marcuse, H. (1976). Repressive tolerance. In P. Connerton (Ed.), *Critical sociology.* Harmondsworth, England: Penguin, pp. 301-329. (Original work published 1965.)

Marx, K. (1977). *Selected writings.* D. McLlellan (Ed.). New York: Oxford University Press.

Marx, K. (1978). Economic and philosophical manuscripts. In R. C. Tucker *The Marx-Engels Reader.* New York: W. W. Norton, pp. 66-125. (Original work published 1844.)

Marx, K. and Engels, F. (1970). *The German ideology.* New York: International Publishers.

McKelvy, D. (1981). Agency change: A response to the needs of Black families and their children. *Child Welfare, 60*(3), 183-190.

Mead, G. H. (1934). *Mind, self, and society.* Edited and with an introduction by Charles W. Morris. Chicago: The University of Chicago Press. Copyright © 1934 by The University of Chicago; Copyright © 1962 by Charles W. Morris, Published 1934, Seventeenth Impression 1970.

Mechanic, D. (1962). Sources of power of lower participants in complex organizations. *Administrative Science Quarterly, 7* (December), 349-364.

Merton, R. K. (1940). Bureaucratic structure and personality. In R. K. Merton, E. P. Gray, B. Hockey, and H. C. Selvin (Eds.). (1952). *Reader in bureaucracy.* New York: Free Press, pp. 361-371.

Miller, D. C. (1992). *Women and social welfare.* New York: Praeger Publishers.

Miller, H. (1981). Dirty sheets: A multi-variate analysis. *Social Work, 26* (July), 268-271.

Mills, C. W. (1961). *The sociological imagination.* New York: Grove Press.

Minors, A. (1995). From uni-versity to poly-versity: Organizations in transition to anti-racism. In C. E. James (Ed.), *Perspectives on racism and the human services sector.* Toronto: University of Toronto Press, pp. 196-208.

Murray, C. (1984). *Losing ground: American social policy 1950-1980.* New York: Basic Books.

Natanson, M. (1967). Phenomenology as a rigorous science. In T. Luckmann (Ed.) (1978). *Phenomenology and sociology.* New York: Penguin, pp. 181-199.

Newdom, F. (1996). Progressive and professional: A contradiction in terms. *BCR Reports, 8.*

Newdom, F. (1997). Guilty your honor, but not guilty enough. *BCR Reports, 9*(1), 1.

Ohlin, L., Piven, H., and Pappenfort, D. (1956). Major dilemmas of the social worker in probation and parole. *The National Probation and Parole Association Journal,* July, 211-225.

The O. M. Collective. (1971). *The organizer's manual.* New York: Bantam Books.

Pease, B. (1997). *Men and sexual politics.* Adelaide, South Australia: Dulwich Centre Publications.

Plato. (1992). Apology. In *The trial and death of Socrates: Four dialogues.* Toronto: General Publishing Company

Prus, R. (1996). *Symbolic interaction and ethnographic research.* Albany, NY: State University of New York.

Rachleff, P. (1993). *Hard-pressed in the heartland: The Hormel strike and the future of the labor movement.* Boston: South End Press.

Racker, H. (1968). *Transference and countertransference.* New York: International Universities Press.

Reamer, F. G. (1995). Ethics and values. In R. L. Edwards and J. G. Hopps (Eds.), *Encyclopedia of Social Work,* Nineteenth edition. Washington: NASW Press, pp. 893-902.

Reeser, L. (1988). Women and social work activism in the 1980's. *Affilia, 3*(3), 51-62.

Reeser, L. and Epstein, I. (1987). Social workers' attitudes toward poverty and social action, 1968-1984. *Social Service Review, 61*(4), 610-622.

Reich, W. (1946). *The mass psychology of fascism.* New York: The Orgone Institute.

Rein, M. (1970). Social work: In search of a radical profession. *Social Work, 15* (2), 13-28.

Rein, M. and White, S. (1981). Knowledge for practice. *Social Service Review, 55*(1), 1-41.

Reisch, M. (1986). From cause to case and back again: The reemergence of advocacy in social work. *Urban and Social Change Review,* Winter/Summer, 20-24.

Reynolds, B. C. (1982). *Between client and community.* Silver Spring, MD: NASW, Inc.

Richan, W. (1988). *Beyond altruism: Social welfare policy in American society.* Binghamton, NY: The Haworth Press.

Richan, W. (1989). Empowering students to empower others. *Journal of Social Work Education, 25*(3), 276-283.

Ricoeur, P. (1970). *Freud and philosophy: An essay on interpretation.* New Haven, CT: Yale University Press.

Roderick, R. (1986). *Habermas and the foundations of critical theory.* New York: St. Martin's Press.

Rycroft, C. (1973). *A critical dictionary of psychoanalysis.* Totowa, NJ: Littlefield Adams.

Sachs, J. (1987) *A social phenomenological investigation of the practice of social work: Toward a fuller understanding and conceptualization of the precipitates of social work practice.* Unpublished dissertation, Adelphi University, Garden City, NY.

Sachs, J. (1989). The therapeutic worth of a client. *Smith College Studies in Social Work, 59,* 146-155.

Sachs, J. (1990). Professionalism, licensure, private practice and the decline of social commitment. *BCRS Reports: Newsletter of the Bertha Capen Reynolds Society, 2*(3-4), 1-5.

Sachs, J. (1991). Action and reflection in work with a group of homeless people. *Social Work with Groups, 14*(3-4), 187-202.

Salomon, A. (1955). *The tyranny of progress.* New York: Noonday Press.

Schutz, A. (1967). *Phenomenology and the social world.* Evanston, IL: Northwestern University Press.

Scotch, R. K. (1988). Disability as the basis for a social movement: Advocacy and the politics of definition. *Journal of Social Issues, 44*(1), 159-172.

Searles, H. F. (1981). The patient as therapist to his analyst. In R. Langs (Ed.), *Classics in psycho-analytic technique.* New York: Jason Aronson, pp. 103-135.

Shor, I. (1996). *When students have power.* Chicago: University of Chicago Press.

Simmel, G. (1950). *The sociology of George Simmel.* New York: Free Press.

Simon, B. (1990). Rethinking empowerment. *Journal of Progressive Human Services, 1*(1), 27-39.

Smelser, N. (1973). *Karl Marx on society and social change.* Chicago: University of Chicago Press.

Stabile, C. S. (1995). Postmodernism, feminism, and Marx: Notes from the abyss. *Monthly Review,* 89-103. Copyright ©1995 by Monthly Review Press. Reprinted by permission of Monthly Review Foundation.

Stein, T. S. and Cohen, C. J. (1986). *Contemporary perspectives on psychotherapy with lesbians and gay men.* New York: Plenum.

Strauss, A. (1956). *George Herbert Mead on social psychology.* Chicago: The University of Chicago Press.

Szasz, T. (1981). The concept of transference. In R. Langs (Ed.), *Classics in psycho-analytic technique.* New York: Jason Aronson, pp. 25-36.

Thomas, W. I. (1967). *The unadjusted girl.* New York: Harper and Row.

Tucker, R. C. (1978). *The Marx-Engels reader.* New York: W. W. Norton.

Walker, P. (1979). *Between labor and capital.* Boston: South End Press.

Weaver, H. N. (1998). Indigenous people in a multicultural society: Unique issues for human services. *Social Work, 43*(3), pp. 203-211.

Weber, M. (1946). *From Max Weber,* H. Gerth and C. W. Mills (Eds.). New York: Oxford University Press.

Weber, M. (1958). *The protestant ethic and the spirit of capitalism* (T. Parsons, Trans.). New York: Charles Scribner and Sons.

Wiggershaus, R. (1994). *The Frankfurt school* (M. Robertson, Trans.). Cambridge, UK: The Polity Press.

Withorn, A. (1986a). For better and for worse: Women against women in the welfare state. In R. Lefkowitz and A. Withorn (Eds.), *For crying out loud.* New York: The Pilgrim Press, pp. 220-234.

Withorn, A. (1986b). What is progressive social work? *Bertha Capen Reynolds Society Newsletter, 1*(2), Fall, 1-2.

Withorn, A. (1996). Professionalism vs. radicalism. *BCR Reports, (8)*2, 1-2.

Wrong, D. (1961). The oversocialized conception of man in modern sociology. *The American Sociological Review, 26*(2), 183-193.

Yevtushenko, Y. (1962). *Selected poems.* Baltimore: Penguin.

Index

Page numbers followed by the letter "i" indicate illustrations.

HAWORTH Social Work Practice
Carlton E. Munson, PhD, Senior Editor

SOCIAL WORK: SEEKING RELEVANCY IN THE TWENTY-FIRST CENTURY by Roland Meinert, John T. Pardeck, and Larry Kreuger. (2000).

SOCIAL WORK PRACTICE IN HOME HEALTH CARE by Ruth Ann Goode. (2000). "Dr. Goode presents both a lucid scenario and a formulated protocol to bring health care services into the home setting. . . . This is a must have volume that will be a reference to be consulted many times." *Marcia B. Steinhauer, PhD, Coordinator and Associate Professor, Human Services Administration Program, Rider University, Lawrenceville, New Jersey*

FORENSIC SOCIAL WORK: LEGAL ASPECTS OF PROFESSIONAL PRACTICE, SECOND EDITION by Robert L. Barker and Douglas M. Branson. (2000). "The authors combine their expertise to create this informative guide to address legal practice issues facing social workers." *Newsletter of the National Organization of Forensic Social Work*

HUMAN SERVICES AND THE AFROCENTRIC PARADIGM by Jerome H. Schiele. (2000). "Represents a milestone in applying the Afrocentric paradigm to human services generally, and social work specifically. . . . A highly valuable resource." *Bogart R. Leashore, PhD, Dean and Professor, Hunter College School of Social Work, New York, New York*

SOCIAL WORK IN THE HEALTH FIELD: A CARE PERSPECTIVE by Lois A. Fort Cowles. (1999). "Makes an important contribution to the field by locating the practice of social work in health care within an organizational and social context." *Goldie Kadushin, PhD, Associate Professor, School of Social Welfare, University of Wisconsin, Milwaukee*

SMART BUT STUCK: WHAT EVERY THERAPIST NEEDS TO KNOW ABOUT LEARNING DISABILITIES AND IMPRISONED INTELLIGENCE by Myrna Orenstein. (1999). "A trailblazing effort that creates an entirely novel way of talking and thinking about learning disabilities. There is simply nothing like it in the field." *Fred M. Levin, MD, Training Supervising Analyst, Chicago Institute for Psychoanalysis; Assistant Professor of Clinical Psychiatry, Northwestern University, School of Medicine, Chicago, IL*

CLINICAL WORK AND SOCIAL ACTION: AN INTEGRATIVE APPROACH by Jerome Sachs and Fred Newdom. (1999). "Just in time for the new millennium come Sachs and Newdom with a wholly fresh look at social work. . . . A much-needed uniting of social work values, theories, and practice for action." *Josephine Nieves, MSW, PhD, Executive Director, National Association of Social Workers*

SOCIAL WORK PRACTICE IN THE MILITARY by James G. Daley. (1999). "A significant and worthwhile book with provocative and stimulating ideas. It deserves to be read by a wide audience in social work education and practice as well as by decision makers in the military." *H. Wayne Johnson, MSW, Professor, University of Iowa, School of Social Work, Iowa City, Iowa*

GROUP WORK: SKILLS AND STRATEGIES FOR EFFECTIVE INTERVENTIONS, SECOND EDITION by Sondra Brandler and Camille P. Roman. (1999). "A clear, basic description of what group work requires, including what skills and techniques group workers need to be effective." *Hospital and Community Psychiatry* (from the first edition)

TEENAGE RUNAWAYS: BROKEN HEARTS AND "BAD ATTITUDES" by Laurie Schaffner (1999). "Skillfully combines the authentic voice of the juvenile runaway with the principles of social science research."

CELEBRATING DIVERSITY: COEXISTING IN A MULTICULTURAL SOCIETY by Benyamin Chetkow-Yanoov. (1999). "Makes a valuable contribution to peace theory and practice." *Ian Harris, EdD, Executive Secretary, Peace Education Committee, International Peace Research Association*

SOCIAL WELFARE POLICY ANALYSIS AND CHOICES by Hobart A. Burch. (1999). "Will become the landmark text in its field for many decades to come." *Sheldon Rahan, DSW, Founding Dean and Emeritus Professor of Social Policy and Social Administration, Faculty of Social Work, Wilfrid Laurier University, Canada*

SOCIAL WORK PRACTICE: A SYSTEMS APPROACH, SECOND EDITION by Benyamin Chetkow-Yannov. (1999). "Highly recommended as a primary text for any and all introductory social work courses." *Ram A. Cnaan, PhD, Associate Professor, School of Social Work, University of Pennsylvania*

CRITICAL SOCIAL WELFARE ISSUES: TOOLS FOR SOCIAL WORK AND HEALTH CARE PROFESSIONALS edited by Arthur J. Katz, Abraham Lurie, and Carlos M. Vidal. (1997). "Offers hopeful agendas for change, while navigating the societal challenges facing those in the human services today." *Book News Inc.*

SOCIAL WORK IN HEALTH SETTINGS: PRACTICE IN CONTEXT, SECOND EDITION edited by Toba Schwaber Kerson. (1997). "A first-class document . . . It will be found among the steadier and lasting works on the social work aspects of American health care." *Hans S. Falck, PhD, Professor Emeritus and Former Chair, Health Specialization in Social Work, Virginia Commonwealth University*

PRINCIPLES OF SOCIAL WORK PRACTICE: A GENERIC PRACTICE APPROACH by Molly R. Hancock. (1997). "Hancock's discussions advocate reflection and self-awareness to create a climate for client change." *Journal of Social Work Education*

NOBODY'S CHILDREN: ORPHANS OF THE HIV EPIDEMIC by Steven F. Dansky. (1997). "Professional sound, moving, and useful for both professionals and interested readers alike." *Ellen G. Friedman, ACSW, Associate Director of Support Services, Beth Israel Medical Center, Methadone Maintenance Treatment Program*

SOCIAL WORK APPROACHES TO CONFLICT RESOLUTION: MAKING FIGHTING OBSOLETE by Benyamin Chetkow-Yanoov. (1996). "Presents an examination of the nature and cause of conflict and suggests techniques for coping with conflict." *Journal of Criminal Justice*

FEMINIST THEORIES AND SOCIAL WORK: APPROACHES AND APPLICATIONS by Christine Flynn Saulnier. (1996). " An essential reference to be read repeatedly by all educators and practitioners who are eager to learn more about feminist theory and practice: *Nancy R. Hooyman, PhD, Dean and Professor, School of Social Work, University of Washington, Seattle*

THE RELATIONAL SYSTEMS MODEL FOR FAMILY THERAPY: LIVING IN THE FOUR REALITIES by Donald R. Bardill. (1996). "Engages the reader in quiet, thoughtful conversation on the timeless issue of helping families and individuals." *Christian Counseling Resource Review*

SOCIAL WORK INTERVENTION IN AN ECONOMIC CRISIS: THE RIVER COMMUNITIES PROJECT by Martha Baum and Pamela Twiss. (1996). "Sets a standard for universities in terms of the types of meaningful roles they can play in supporting and sustaining communities." *Kenneth J. Jaros, PhD, Director, Public Health Social Work Training Program, University of Pittsburgh*

FUNDAMENTALS OF COGNITIVE-BEHAVIOR THERAPY: FROM BOTH SIDES OF THE DESK by Bill Borcherdt. (1996). "Both beginning and experienced practitioners . . . will find a considerable number of valuable suggestions in Borcherdt's book." *Albert Ellis, PhD, President, Institute for Rational-Emotive Therapy, New York City*

BASIC SOCIAL POLICY AND PLANNING: STRATEGIES AND PRACTICE METHODS by Hobart A. Burch. (1996). "Burch's familiarity with his topic is evident and his book is an easy introduction to the field." *Readings*

THE CROSS-CULTURAL PRACTICE OF CLINICAL CASE MANAGEMENT IN MENTAL HEALTH edited by Peter Manoleas. (1996). "Makes a contribution by bringing together the cross-cultural and clinical case management perspectives in working with those who have serious mental illness." *Disability Studies Quarterly*

FAMILY BEYOND FAMILY: THE SURROGATE PARENT IN SCHOOLS AND OTHER COMMUNITY AGENCIES by Sanford Weinstein. (1995). "Highly recommended to anyone concerned about the welfare of our children and the breakdown of the American family." *Jerold S. Greenberg, EdD, Director of Community Service, College of Health & Human Performance, University of Maryland*

PEOPLE WITH HIV AND THOSE WHO HELP THEM: CHALLENGES, INTEGRATION, INTERVENTION by R. Dennis Shelby. (1995). "A useful and compassionate contribution to the HIV psychotherapy literature." *Public Health*

THE BLACK ELDERLY: SATISFACTION AND QUALITY OF LATER LIFE by Marguerite Coke and James A. Twaite. (1995). "Presents a model for predicting life satisfaction in this population." *Abstracts in Social Gerontology*

BUILDING ON WOMEN'S STRENGTHS: A SOCIAL WORK AGENDA FOR THE TWENTY-FIRST CENTURY edited by Liane V. Davis. (1994). "The most lucid and accessible overview of the related epistemological debates int he social work literature." *Journal of the National Association of Social Workers*

NOW DARE EVERYTHING: TALES OF HIV-RELATED PSYCHOTHERAPY by Steven F. Dansky. (1994). "A highly recommended book for anyone working with persons who are HIV positive. . . . Every library should have a copy of this book." *AIDS Book Review Journal*

INTERVENTION RESEARCH: DESIGN AND DEVELOPMENT FOR HUMAN SERVICE edited by Jack Rothman and Edwin J. Thomas. (1994). "Provides a useful framework for the further examination of methodology for each separate step of such research." *Academic Library Book Review*

CLINICAL SOCIAL WORK SUPERVISION, SECOND EDITION by Carlton E. Munson. (1993). "A useful, thorough, and articulate reference for supervisors and for 'supervisees' who are wanting to understand their supervisor or are looking for effective supervision." *Transactional Analysis Journal*

ELEMENTS OF THE HELPING PROCESS: A GUIDE FOR CLINICIANS by Raymond Fox. (1993). "Filled with helpful hints, creative interventions, and practical guidelines." *Journal of Family Psychotherapy*

IF A PARTNER HAS AIDS: GUIDE TO CLINICAL INTERVENTION FOR RELATIONSHIPS IN CRISIS by R. Dennis Shelby. (1993). " A welcome addition to existing publications about couples coping with AIDS, it offers intervention ideas and strategies to clinicians." *Contemporary Psychology*

GERONTOLOGICAL SOCIAL WORK SUPERVISION by Ann Burack-Weiss and Frances Coyle Brennan. (1991). "The creative ideas in this book will aid supervisors working with students and experienced social workers." *Senior News*

SOCIAL WORK THEORY AND PRACTICE WITH THE TERMINALLY ILL by Joan K. Parry. (1989). "Should be read by all professionals engaged in the provision of health services in hospitals, emergency rooms, and hospices." *Hector B. Garcia, PhD, Professor, San Jose State University School of Social Work*

THE CREATIVE PRACTITIONER: THEORY AND METHODS FOR THE HELPING SERVICES by Bernard Gelfand. (1988). "[Should] be widely adopted by those in the helping services. It could lead to significant positive advances by countless individuals." *Sidney J. Parnes, Trustee Chairperson for Strategic Program Development, Creative Education Foundation, Buffalo, NY*

MANAGEMENT AND INFORMATION SYSTEMS IN HUMAN SERVICES: IMPLICATIONS FOR THE DISTRIBUTION OF AUTHORITY AND DECISION MAKING by Richard K. Caputo. (1987). "A contribution to social work scholarship in that it provides conceptual frameworks that can be used in the design of management information systems." *Social Work*

Order Your Own Copy of
This Important Book for Your Personal Library!

CLINICAL WORK AND SOCIAL ACTION
An Integrative Approach

_____ in hardbound at $39.95 (ISBN:0-7890-0278-7)

_____ in softbound at $24.95 (ISBN: 0-7890-0279-5)

COST OF BOOKS_____

OUTSIDE USA/CANADA/
MEXICO: ADD 20%_____

POSTAGE & HANDLING_____
(US: $3.00 for first book & $1.25
for each additional book)
Outside US: $4.75 for first book
& $1.75 for each additional book)

SUBTOTAL_____

IN CANADA: ADD 7% GST_____

STATE TAX_____
(NY, OH & MN residents, please
add appropriate local sales tax)

FINAL TOTAL_____
(If paying in Canadian funds,
convert using the current
exchange rate. UNESCO
coupons welcome.)

☐ **BILL ME LATER:** ($5 service charge will be added)
(Bill-me option is good on US/Canada/Mexico orders only;
not good to jobbers, wholesalers, or subscription agencies.)

☐ Check here if billing address is different from
shipping address and attach purchase order and
billing address information.

Signature_____

☐ **PAYMENT ENCLOSED: $**_____

☐ **PLEASE CHARGE TO MY CREDIT CARD.**

☐ Visa   ☐ MasterCard   ☐ AmEx   ☐ Discover
☐ Diners Club
Account #_____

Exp. Date_____

Signature_____

Prices in US dollars and subject to change without notice.

NAME_____

INSTITUTION_____

ADDRESS_____

CITY_____

STATE/ZIP_____

COUNTRY_____ COUNTY (NY residents only)_____

TEL_____ FAX_____

E-MAIL_____
May we use your e-mail address for confirmations and other types of information? ☐ Yes   ☐ No

Order From Your Local Bookstore or Directly From
The Haworth Press, Inc.
10 Alice Street, Binghamton, New York 13904-1580 • USA
TELEPHONE: 1-800-HAWORTH (1-800-429-6784) / Outside US/Canada: (607) 722-5857
FAX: 1-800-895-0582 / Outside US/Canada: (607) 772-6362
E-mail: getinfo@haworthpressinc.com
PLEASE PHOTOCOPY THIS FORM FOR YOUR PERSONAL USE.

BOF96